WHY
BREASTFEEDING
GRIEF AND TRAUMA
MATTER

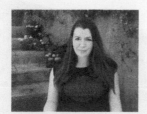

About the author

Professor Amy Brown is based in the Department of Public Health, Policy and Social Sciences at Swansea University in the UK, where she leads the MSc in Child Public Health. With a background in psychology, she first became interested in the many barriers women face when breastfeeding after having her first baby. Three babies and a PhD later she has spent the last 12 years exploring psychological, cultural and societal barriers to breastfeeding, with an emphasis on understanding how we can better support women to breastfeed and subsequently raise breastfeeding rates. Her primary focus is how we can shift our perception of breastfeeding as an individual mothering issue, to a wider public health responsibility, with consideration of how we can make societal changes to protect and encourage breastfeeding.

Professor Brown has published over 100 papers exploring the barriers women face in feeding their baby during the first year. In 2016 she published her first book *Breastfeeding Uncovered*, followed by *Why Starting Solids Matters* (2017), *The Positive Breastfeeding Book* (2018), *Informed is Best* and *Why Breastfeeding Grief and Trauma Matter* (both 2019), *Let's talk about the first year of parenting* (2020), and *Let's talk about feeding your baby* (2021).

She is a regular blogger, aiming to change the way we think about breastfeeding, mothering and caring for our babies.

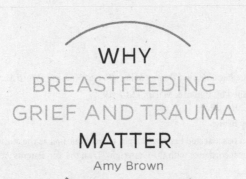

WHY
BREASTFEEDING
GRIEF AND TRAUMA
MATTER

Amy Brown

pinter
&
martin

Why Breastfeeding Grief and Trauma Matter (Pinter & Martin Why It Matters 17)

First published by Pinter & Martin Ltd 2019
Reprinted 2021, 2023

ISBN 978-1-78066-615-0

Also available as an ebook

Pinter & Martin Why It Matters ISSN 2056-8657
Series editor: Susan Last
Index: Helen Bilton

British Library Cataloguing-in-Publication Data

A catalogue record for this book is available from the British Library.

Set in Minion

Printed and bound in the UK by Clays

This book has been printed on paper that is sourced and harvested from sustainable forests and is FSC accredited.

Pinter & Martin Ltd
6 Effra Parade
London SW2 1PS

pinterandmartin.com

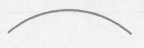

Contents

You did not fail.

No woman 'fails' to breastfeed.

They are failed by a system that fails to support them,
both during breastfeeding and when they cannot.

And that is what we are going to change.

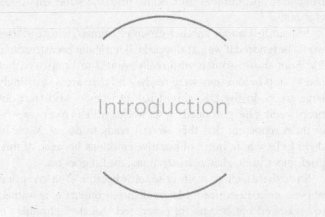

Introduction

How often do you look at a newspaper or social media headline and see yet another story about how there is 'too much pressure' on women to breastfeed, and that this pressure from health professionals and 'lactivists' leaves women feeling guilty and miserable? The implication is that we should stop going on about breastfeeding, because talking about it makes women who couldn't do it feel bad.

Is stopping talking about breastfeeding really the answer? Or is it more complex than that?

We are of course all different. Some women want to formula feed their baby from the start. Some have no real preference, so they give breastfeeding a go but aren't bothered if it doesn't work out. That is great. But those aren't the women this book is about.

Others may have only tried to breastfeed because they felt they 'should', reporting they felt pressure from others to breastfeed. This is a complex issue, deeply embedded in the way in which society tries to control women by judging their behaviour and choices. But again, this isn't what this book is about.

Instead it is about another group of women, whose stories would be ignored if we just stopped talking about breastfeeding. It's about those women who really *wanted* to breastfeed but had to stop before they were ready. And they are a startlingly large group. In the UK, almost half of women who start out breastfeeding have stopped by six weeks, with as many as 90% of them reporting that they weren't ready to do so. Many of them feel a whole range of negative emotions because of this: grief, anger, guilt, shame, frustration... the list goes on.

So do these feelings really arise solely because of a perception of 'pressure' to breastfeed? Maybe all these women never wanted to breastfeed but because of others feel that they should? Or could it be that many women's feelings about how they feed their babies run much deeper?

How a woman feels when she wants to breastfeed but cannot can be much more complicated than simply the idea she is being made to feel guilty by others. When women who couldn't breastfeed talk to me, often about babies who are now grown up, their emotions come tumbling out. There's the guilt, yes. But also grief. And anger. Trauma. Anxiety. With frustration, isolation and failure added in for good measure. They talk about loss. The loss of a particular relationship with their baby. The loss of a way of mothering. The loss of how they saw themselves.

It is fair to say that many are grieving.

Where is all this emotion in the headlines? It is, of course, not there. Instead, headlines, designed to be sensational, insist that breastfeeding doesn't really matter to women, and that breastfeeding support is all just part of some big 'lactivist agenda'. The articles don't stop to consider the idea that maybe women want to breastfeed for their own reasons. They don't ask why women in the UK and USA, for example, seem to struggle more with breastfeeding than women in many other countries. They don't do anything to try to fix the situation so that more women can breastfeed.

They just blame. And minimise. And deflect. Consequently making the situation even worse for future generations of women, or for those in marginalised groups who need the protection of breastfeeding the most. It's time we stopped the debate and focused on the future: a future in which all women have the infant feeding support they need without question.

It's also time we recognised why supporting breastfeeding is so important. Yes, it matters because on a population level it affects the health of our future generations. But for once, this isn't what we're focusing on. In fact, this book is barely going to mention babies at all. Instead, it's about women's reproductive rights, and enabling them to mother through breastfeeding in the way they want. It's about recognising the emotional impact not breastfeeding can have on women and helping them heal. And most importantly of all it's about making sure we change things for the next generation of mothers, so they don't experience this pain.

Three years ago I put out a research request asking women to describe how they felt if they were unable to breastfeed for as long as they wanted and felt negatively about that. Over 2,000 women responded within a week. This book tells their story, and explains why we should all care about supporting women, however they feed their babies.

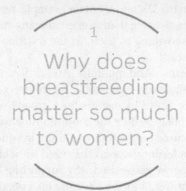

1

Why does breastfeeding matter so much to women?

Warning: this chapter considers all the ways in which breastfeeding is important to women, considering what they lose over and above just being able to give their baby milk. It considers breastfeeding in the context of it being a woman's reproductive right, and the ways in which breastfeeding can enhance a woman's life or is otherwise important to her, for example for religious, spiritual and cultural reasons.

It is vitally important that we discuss this fully, as a belief that breastfeeding is just about nutrition harms women by telling them that their experiences do not matter. It is vital that others learn about what breastfeeding can mean. It is not good enough to tell women that none of their feelings matter as long as their baby is fed, and that they can just give a bottle instead.

However, if you are currently in despair about not being able to breastfeed you may wish to approach this chapter with caution. Some women have told me that reading about how important breastfeeding is can be cathartic, and that they feel understood and validated. But for others it is too difficult, and that is fair enough. So if you're feeling like this, please, skip to the next chapter.

So why does breastfeeding matter so much to women? I mean, isn't it just a way of getting milk into a baby? What's wrong with the message *'Give it a go, and if you can't then formula is nutritionally complete, so just give a bottle. The main thing is your baby is fed – now go and get on with it.'*?

Every mother out there surely agrees that the main thing is that their baby is fed. And they can feel grateful that they have the option of formula milk, when generations ago many babies who could not have breastmilk would have died or become malnourished due to inadequate diets. For some mothers, their breastfeeding journey ends quite happily here – happy they tried, disappointed it didn't work, but content to bottle-feed formula.

For others, the story is more complex. For them, breastfeeding wasn't just about milk, it was so much more. And there are many ways in which breastfeeding isn't just about nutrition, but also about things like mothering, healing and history.

Before we look at all the different ways in which breastfeeding matters to women, I want to make one thing very clear. Some women want to breastfeed. Others do not. Some feel okay when they can't, while others describe this experience as nothing short of devastating. There is no one right way to feel. Caring about breastfeeding doesn't in any way make women 'better' mothers, it just means that for them, breastfeeding was important. It isn't a judgement on others who do not want to breastfeed. Nor is caring about breastfeeding and feeling it to be part of your identity making it 'all about you'. As we'll see, men are allowed to feel that their bodily autonomy is an important part of their identity. Everyone recognises this and thinks it's very important to do research and support them, while simultaneously mocking and criticising women for doing the same.

With that out of the way, let's look at why breastfeeding matters to women.

Is it because of its impact on babies' health?

If you ask women why they wanted to breastfeed, the response many will automatically give is often based around how human milk helps protect babies' health and development. I mean, that's what we're told is important, isn't it? Most health promotion campaigns tell you that breastfeeding is a good idea because it helps reduce how many colds or stomach bugs babies get.

And yes, that's very important. When women can't breastfeed one of their main concerns is that their baby will be harmed by not being breastfed. They wanted to increase their baby's protection against illness, particularly if their baby was born sick or too soon. As mothers, parents, human beings, we worry about and want the best for our babies.

But this is not the only reason why breastfeeding matters. Many women who cannot breastfeed find that their baby is indeed 'fine' when they move to formula milk, as breastfeeding is not actually a miracle elixir that can stop every single illness in its tracks. Nor does not breastfeeding automatically doom your baby to a lifetime of poor health. Health is complicated and affected by lots of things. But just because her baby is 'fine', doesn't mean a woman is fine. Breastfeeding is more than trying to beat the health odds.

My story – Jane Woodley

I breastfeed my babies. It's what I know. It's how I do mothering. My first two sons, born 21 months apart in 2004 and 2006, were breastfed for 18 months and four years respectively. I've supported many other women to breastfeed their babies. I've had writing published about breastfeeding, I've spoken publicly about it.

My third son was born in 2017, four and a bit weeks premature. Having been used to 8lb+ term plus babies, this tiny 5lb 4oz bundle was a surprise addition to the family in more ways than just his early entrance. I was diabetic when I was pregnant with him, so I'd started to hand-express colostrum to freeze in little syringes. When it became clear that he didn't have much in the way of a rooting reflex and wasn't opening his mouth to latch, he got through all I could produce and still his blood sugars weren't good. I'd had no sleep for 48 hours, an induced labour and was hallucinating husky dogs in Norwegian forests and pulsating rainbow owls. He had a bit of formula and I wept, slept and regrouped. Then I asked for the breast pump and so began a journey into the heady world of exclusive pumping. Spoiler alert: glamorous it ain't.

We were discharged from hospital after eight days. Long story short – he was diagnosed with tongue tie after 11 weeks of expressing, very occasional latching and bottle logistics I'd never had to contend with before as a breastfeeding mum. He had his tongue tie snipped by a private lactation consultant (IBCLC), but he still couldn't latch (one London NHS clinic had wanted him to be 'breastfeeding confidently four times a day' to carry it out, which I felt was like expecting someone to be running the 100 metres before they could qualify for a wheelchair. And an appointment at a different clinic was still a couple of months away). The night before the IBCLC came back for a follow-up visit was my nadir. I finished my last express of the day and went through the ritual of sorting the milk and pump parts out for the middle of the night feed and pump session.

I lay next to him, fast asleep in our bedroom, and tried to tell myself that his tummy was full of my milk, that his body was growing and filling out as a result of my efforts with expressing. Was I being selfish, wanting the breastfeeding experience solely for myself? He was happy, so why couldn't I be? But I knew – I knew what it was like to latch my child and feed them till they were milk-drunk, their starfish hands grasping then patting then quiet, feeling them calm and relax into me. And, further on, I knew what it was like to feed a toddler, the reassuring comfort it gives them when the world and their emotions are just too big, the 'fill in the diet gaps' nutrition breastmilk provides.

Wanting him to be breastfed wasn't just about me, not by a long way. And, whatever I tried to tell myself, pumping my milk and it being either my husband or me who fed him from a bottle wasn't the same. And he was gulpy, windy, possetty – it wasn't comfortable for him either. I'd been torturing myself, reading articles about how much better for a baby's immune system it was to feed directly than to express. But how much longer could I keep expressing? The constant worrying about producing enough, diligently noting down how much I was producing each day, how much he'd taken, was I staying far enough ahead of his needs, what about the next growth spurt? At some point, I knew it was likely I would have to introduce formula.

We were gearing up for World Breastfeeding Week, Mark Zuckerberg was about to have a new baby and everyone was posting about breastfeeding selfies or 'brelfies'. Social media seemed to be full of happy mums whose babies latched beautifully. I felt cheated, resentful, guilty that I hadn't pushed harder to work out why my newest little lad couldn't latch. I'd accepted the hospital's reasoning that he was just too little and he'd learn as he got bigger.

But, mostly, I just felt sad, more than sad – I felt like I was grieving. And, having immersed myself in the world of breastfeeding support and thought at length about how to help women to breastfeed, I felt like I never wanted to hear the word again, much less have anything to do with anyone who still inhabited that world. I didn't want the reminder that, this time, the oh-so-natural process just wasn't working, that my dear little baby was being so thoroughly failed by his mother. If I couldn't breastfeed and expressing was likely to get more difficult both logistically and in terms of production as my son got older, more mobile and spent more time awake – what could I do? Intellectually, I knew that formula wasn't likely to harm him, but when he'd had some in hospital, he smelt wrong – not like my baby. I felt utterly wretched and so, so stuck.

Feeding had become a simple transaction: empty baby plus full bottle equals full baby. And it wasn't a transaction I wanted; it was a relationship. Because, for me, breastfeeding wasn't just about getting milk into my baby. It was so much more than that; it was the quiet moments holding my baby in my arms at the end of the day, the cheeky trying to talk with their mouth full, mischief eyes looking up at me, the patting to say which side they wanted first, sitting up post-feed and saying, 'Yum!' and all the other skin-on-skin moments that were so important for bonding. None of these little snapshots of mothering included a hospital-grade breast pump and bottles, though I was incredibly grateful both things existed. But I was heartbroken, grieving my lost relationship.

The next day, after a two-hour session with the IBCLC that included nipple shields, bottle teats and a supplemental nursing system (SNS), along with much expressed milk and position switching, he finally latched and fed for 25 minutes. Over the course of the next couple of days, we managed to drop the SNS as he learnt that there would be milk once he'd latched and sucked a few times. And, some two years later, having just tucked him into bed after his bedtime breastfeed, it feels like a different lifetime.

But I will never forget how close I came to needing a different narrative to get me through what was an extremely difficult time. And I am now fascinated by just how difficult and painful I found reading or hearing anything about breastfeeding when I didn't think it was going to work for us this time.

Jane's story tells us so much about why breastfeeding is more than just milk and why so many women go to such efforts to desperately try to make it work when the odds are stacked against them. It's about mothering and comfort and instinct. It is something deep, instinctual and automatic. A decision that many women don't consciously make – they just want to do it.[1] In fact, why on earth would you even ask the question? We don't for any other bodily function… Tell me, sir, when did you make the decision that you wanted to walk?

All of this means that one of the biggest emotions women can feel when they can't breastfeed is *shock*. Shock that it isn't working. Shock that there seem to be no answers. Shock that no one really seems to care.

Breastfeeding as a reproductive and bodily right

Breastfeeding, on one level, is one of the most basic of all bodily functions. It has sustained generations and generations of babies. The early stages of breastmilk are produced automatically; at first during pregnancy and then in larger amounts once the placenta is out. From then on milk is produced in response to milk being removed from the breasts: the more milk that is removed, the more that is made to replace it. But at first, it is an automatic response of the body. This is not to be confused with biological determinism. Just because women are 'designed' to produce milk after birth, does not mean they are required to use that milk from a sociocultural perspective. However, at birth, their body has not recognised that wider social context, and prepares for a baby to be fed.[2]

Breastfeeding is closely tied to maternal reproductive and physical health. Not breastfeeding is associated with an increased risk of reproductive cancers, heart disease, diabetes and weight gain. Breastfeeding protects women physiologically from the stress of motherhood, enhancing sleep, reducing stress and downregulating inflammation, resulting in better mental health (more on this later). Meanwhile, breastfeeding delays the return of ovulation after birth – which means a usually welcome delay in the return of periods for women in more privileged societies, and the ability to space children and protect their own health and even life for women without access to contraception and healthcare.[3] If this was all available in a 'pill' its inventor would be richer than their wildest dreams, lauded as a saviour of maternal health. How dare we tell women it just doesn't matter if they can't breastfeed?

When breastfeeding goes wrong, many women find that isn't even queried by the medical profession. They are told they can't breastfeed and to simply give a bottle instead, as if breastfeeding was just about a way of getting milk into a baby rather than a function of their body. They may be very relieved to have the option of formula milk in these circumstances. But that doesn't mean it's a simple swap. If you have hearing loss, you're likely very grateful for your hearing aid, but no one would expect you not to care about your loss of bodily function. No one dismisses your feelings by telling you that the main thing that matters is that you can hear, so you should just get on with it. Yet we see this message time and time again with breastfeeding.

And with breastfeeding, many women don't even get a diagnosis. When you suddenly lose your hearing, the medical profession doesn't simply say 'Oh, that's a shame, buy a hearing aid'; there will be tests and explorations and an attempt to work out *why*. But where are the tests and diagnoses for women who can't breastfeed? Where is the branch of medicine specialising in lactation issues?

Compare this with a male sexual organ dysfunction: erectile dysfunction (inability to obtain or sustain an erection). Although this involves a primary rather than a secondary sexual characteristic, sufferers are never told that their loss of function does not matter. Investment in research and treatment for the condition is considerable, with nine billion dollars spent globally on prescriptions each year.[4] Five times as much research is conducted into erectile dysfunction than into premenstrual syndrome and dysphoric disorder, despite this affecting five times more women.[5] Male bodily dysfunction is recognised as significant, important and worth investing in. There is research into its origins, treatment and psychological impact on men and their identity.[6] But breastfeeding? Just give a bottle... the main thing is your baby is fed... don't be ridiculous.

Breastfeeding is a way of mothering

Critics of breastfeeding can get angry at the idea that for some women, breastfeeding is an important part of their maternal identity,[7] but mothering and breastfeeding go hand in hand for many. It is also the very image of motherhood – after all, many famous paintings and statues depict a mother with a baby at her breast (my personal favourite being the Fountain of Neptune in Bologna – if you haven't seen it, google it immediately!). This is not to say that breastfeeding is about being a 'good' mother or not, or that you're not really a mother if you don't breastfeed. But many women feel that breastfeeding is consciously or subconsciously bound up with their desired image of mothering.

Breastfeeding is so much more than milk delivery. It is a way to calm, soothe and distract a baby. In this way, breastfeeding also leads to bonding and closeness. Again, this is not to say that breastfeeding is the *only* way in which mothers can bond, but it is most certainly one of the ways. Oxytocin levels – which promote feelings of calmness, closeness and togetherness – rise in both mother and baby during breastfeeding. Mothers feel connected to their babies, and experience a great sense of intimacy.[8] So when mothers are no longer able to breastfeed, they're not only losing the physical milk transfer, but also the way of mothering they wanted to have. They grieve – for the loss of breastfeeding, and also the image of the mother they envisaged themselves to be.

Breastfeeding – dare I say it – is such a convenient way of mothering once you've got the hang of it. Society hates the idea of mothers having anything to benefit them, but many mothers say that once they get past those early weeks, and get into a rhythm of breastfeeding, then breastfeeding feels like the easier option. No planning or forgetting. And little money to pay out (this is not to be confused with breastfeeding having no value – it does, women's time is worth phenomenal amounts).

When breastfeeding starts to go wrong, it is the opposite of easy. Breastfeeding difficulties are time-consuming, both practically and emotionally. It can start to cost large amounts of money in appointments and stuff you hope will help. And then, if it doesn't get better, women lose even more. Gone is the convenience and in its place comes forward planning and logistics. This is invariably even more difficult for women already in stressful situations. When you're living in poverty, dealing with an illness or disability yourself, or have lots of other children and caring responsibilities, breastfeeding can make all the difference. And it's okay for women to grieve this added work.

Breastfeeding can be a way of healing

Breastfeeding can also be a healer, particularly for mothers who have had a difficult birth or whose baby is sick or premature. Some women report that although they felt their body 'let them down' during birth, with labour not going the way they hoped, being able to breastfeed helped them see their body differently. It worked again, like it 'should'.

For mothers with a baby in special care, being able to feed them, or express milk for them, can help in so many ways. They might feel that they have 'failed' their baby because they were born sick or too soon (again, of course they have not), but being able to give their milk to their baby to help them grow and get stronger makes them feel that their body is working again.[9] For those with a baby who is wired up to different machines, and where nurses and doctors seem to be in charge, breastfeeding and giving breastmilk can help parents feel that they are 'reclaiming' their baby for themselves. This is especially true if they are able to hold their baby, away from the machines.[10]

Of course, when breastfeeding then doesn't work out after a difficult birth (and a difficult birth can mean it's less likely to work out, as we'll see later on), then feelings of 'failure' can be compounded and exacerbated. Already battered physically and emotionally by a difficult birth, mothers then have to process struggling to breastfeed, often knowing that this is a direct consequence of their birth. If mothers struggle to feed or express milk, precisely because their baby was born too soon, the trauma can instead be exacerbated, compounded by the feeling of urgency of their tiny, sick baby needing their milk.

Of course, it is not just tiny babies who are sick and can benefit from being 'nursed' through their illness. When older children get sick, breastfeeding can be a lifeline for them, both in terms of delivering key nutrients and also as a comfort, pain reliever and way of connecting. As Lyndsey Hookway, IBCLC writes:

I've always been passionate about breastfeeding. I never set a time limit on it, and never consciously thought about breastfeeding a preschooler. But its importance was brought into sharp focus when my second child developed sepsis, and was then diagnosed with cancer. To be honest, at the age of 3.5 years, I was actually hoping she would stop. But when your child is critically ill, everything changes. I'm grateful of course to advances in chemotherapy which have undoubtedly saved my daughter's life. But there have been times over the last 26 months of treatment when breastfeeding meant the world.

It was why she never had a nasogastric tube when she suffered from the toxic side effects of her high-dose chemo and couldn't eat for two weeks. It eased her nausea. It helped when even morphine didn't touch the pain. It was why she never suffered from painful mouth and gastric ulcers that we were warned about.

It was her connection to normal. It was my reminder of the importance of relationship, responsiveness and comfort. I can't prove it, but I credit breastfeeding for the maintenance of her joyful character and resilience through all the awfulness, and comparative wellness during severe immune suppression. Breastfeeding for us was almost nothing to do with nutrition, and everything to do with everything else.

Breastfeeding and healing is also not just about sick babies and children. It can be about a woman healing her own traumas through having power over her body again. Although not all women will feel this way, some women who have had eating disorders have talked about how breastfeeding helps them see their body in a new light – a stronger and more meaningful light. One woman with a history of anorexia and bulimia explained:

I remember hating my body since I was about 4 and feeling like I needed to punish myself through punishing it. My main thoughts about my body were all about how I was going to binge and purge and hurt it (and alternatively try to starve it). When my daughter was born I didn't really mean to breastfeed but thought I would give her a feed and something in me just clicked. I was using my body in a positive way and she was literally thriving in front of me, growing bigger and stronger. She was such a happy baby and I wonder if it helped connect everything. I'm not fully healed and not sure I ever will be, but my experience of breastfeeding her helped me to start seeing my body in a different, more powerful and useful way.

Breastfeeding can also be a way of healing for survivors of sexual abuse. Although for some breastfeeding will remind them of the trauma, for others it can feel like they are reclaiming their body by using it to breastfeed and nourish a baby. It can be a symbol of feminine power if you felt your power was lost to a man. It can be a symbol of control. You are choosing to breastfeed. You are creating positive memories with your body that will have a lifelong positive impact. Your breasts are the focus for nutrition, not sex. Research has even shown that among mothers with a history of sexual abuse, although sleep difficulties and depression were high in the sample, those who were breastfeeding had fewer issues, likely because of the protective hormonal effect of breastfeeding.[11]

Breastfeeding may also help mothers heal from other physical harm. Survivors of female genital mutilation, for example, have described how breastfeeding helped them overcome some of the hurt, through being able to use their body in the way it was intended. As one Somali mother put it:

Breastfeeding mattered so much to me because as a young girl having gone through FGM a part of me was taken away in the most traumatic and indiscriminate way. Breastfeeding was something that involved a part of the female anatomy and that was something I had control over and was able to empower myself through it by breastfeeding my children. Many Somali woman find breastfeeding very important because it allows them to regain control of their body and what it's for. Being a survivor of FGM has made me more aware of what I need to reclaim as mine and yes, breastfeeding has helped me overcome a lot things as well as helped me feel empowered and complete as woman. It may sound weird but breastfeeding did compensate for what I felt I lost as a child.

Last but not least, breastfeeding can be a way of healing from emotional trauma, especially the intergenerational, historical type. I spoke with Chimine Arfuso, PhD (ABD), an expert in intergenerational trauma and breastfeeding:

If we consider the impact of trauma on breastfeeding from a multi-generational lens, whether or not a mother herself was breastfed, or if her mother was breastfed, breastfeeding becomes an oral tradition or birthrite that is entangled with sociological and political histories. When looking at it from this perspective, we now see how family migration patterns and the trauma associated with these migrations, such as being a refugee, a descendant of the transatlantic slave diaspora, a descendent of a Holocaust survivor, immigration, etc, can impact breastfeeding relationships for generations to come.

Epigenetics have shown that trauma can be inherited. Imagine a trauma your grandmother experienced while five months pregnant with your mother, when the egg that would one day make you was present and already fully formed. To use myself as an example, when my grandmother was pregnant with my mother, they lived in Cuba pre-revolution; however, my mother was only a few months old when Fidel successfully overthrew Baptista in Cuba. Therefore, any political anxiety or unrest with revolution my grandmother experienced while pregnant with my mother, was passed down to me while my mother was in my grandmother's womb.

For women of colour and other marginalised communities, it is possible to start to repair these histories of trauma through a reclamation of breastfeeding as an oral tradition. Additionally, from a neurological brain perspective, breastfeeding, but more specifically eye synchronicity (the deep eye-gazing that occurs naturally with the close contact required in the breastfeeding relationship) can actually begin to rewire trauma connections in the brain. Additionally, we are learning more and more about how crucial pregnancy and early post-partum is for mothers in brain development and as a time in which there is a larger capacity to heal trauma in the brain.

Breastfeeding is tied to culture

Breastfeeding is deeply embedded in the culture and history of many women. It can be part of who they and their community are, a behaviour that is synonymous with motherhood and being a mother in that particular community. It is not just part of individual identity, but community and cultural identity. It can also be about reclaiming cultural identity.

This is particularly true for communities around the world who have had their history and rights taken away through practices such as colonialism, dispersal and slavery. Being able to breastfeed is a powerful way of reclaiming history and traditions and connecting with ancestors. For example, as Camie Goldhammer, clinical social worker, IBCLC and Indigenous Breastfeeding Advocate, described:

> *When we frame breastfeeding not as a feeding choice, but a cultural or traditional practice, we are forced to look at the impact of colonialism and its role in the loss of breastfeeding in Indigenous communities. When Indigenous people breastfeed their babies they are reclaiming their traditional practices, which not only has the power to change the life course of future generations, but heal those that came before us.*

Speaking about breastfeeding and black women in the US, Kimberly Seals Allers, journalist, maternal and infant health strategist, and author of *The Big Letdown: How Medicine, Big Business and Feminism Undermine Breastfeeding*, explains the importance of being able to breastfeed on so many levels:

> *Black breastfeeding is a revolutionary act, an act of resistance in and of itself. When black women breastfeed, they are*

reversing narratives, reclaiming traditions that were taken from them, countering stereotypes and reestablishing the infant feeding norm in our communities. For black women, breastfeeding creates sisterhood and community as we develop peer models of support where larger systems have failed us.

There can be no conversation about the landscape of black breastfeeding in the US without a foundational conversation about the impact of racism and class on breastfeeding rates. In the US the historical context and structural oppression is clear: during slavery black women were often forced to stop breastfeeding their own children to breastfeed the children of their slave owners. This led to a corruption and a disruption of the maternal bond and infant feeding relationship. Later, as cultural norms about white motherhood changed, black and brown women were primarily used as wet nurses – often this being one of few forms of paid labour they could access.

The legacy and historical trauma of this disruption lingers today where in the US significant racial disparities in breastfeeding rates have persisted for over 40 years. Those historical forces have been aided and abetted by disparities in support. For example, in the US, the premier breastfeeding support organisation, La Leche League, which has been on the frontiers of mother-led advocacy and support for breastfeeding, has traditionally been located in white suburban areas and focused on stay-at-home mothers. Women of colour have traditionally worked outside the home, creating pockets of support around white women and leaving women of colour and working women on their own. When white women are centred in how breastfeeding support is designed and located, then women of colour continue to pay the price.

Black breastfeeding, and important awareness campaigns such as Black Breastfeeding Week are a declaration that we as black mothers will not settle for a manufactured artificial food substance that is aggressively peddled particularly in our communities. We will not give in to being sold on the message that we should settle for 'good enough.' We will not quickly give in to the corporate influences and profit-making interests that want us to feed our babies synthetic food from birth and then flood our communities with poor food options and targeted cigarette advertising. We are eyes wide open to the system that from day one of life wants to give our babies less than, give our schools less than, give our communities less than, then treat our young men as less than.

Breastfeeding is our living, breathing, lactating, sucking and nurturing rallying sign against the norm. A personal protest sign (fist up, breast out). It is about us reclaiming our bodies from the media world, from the hyper-sexualised images and from the hip-hop culture, and feeling empowered to execute our biological norm for the benefit of our babies. And it's about our men having our backs as we do so. And as we are demanding systemic change in our communities, the black breastfeeding movement is also about us insisting on having the same breastfeeding support systems that gladly go into white affluent neighbors but somehow avoid our neighbourhoods. It means we can and will create our own. It is about demanding more from physicians and other healthcare professionals who don't bother to educate us or our husbands and partners about breastfeeding because they've assumed we won't do it anyway. Or they don't trust us to do it right.

It is a statement that our babies matter. Their health matters. Our health matters. Our lives matter. Breastfeeding is the beginning of changing our narrative.

In the UK, although the history of breastfeeding and ethnicity is different from the US, breastfeeding is still of particular importance for women of colour. First, the protection of breastfeeding for maternal and infant health is important to help reduce the shocking racially driven disparities women of colour experience even in a rich country such as the UK. Second, breastfeeding can still very much be tied to the identity of black women. It is part of history and tradition. Anna Horn, a breastfeeding specialist and postnatal doula who runs Every Woman Doula in the UK, explained:

> *The motivations that drive women to breastfeed are not just limited to health and the wellbeing of the baby. Often women from black African backgrounds, for example, are aware of the normality of breastfeeding in their ancestral homes and wish to practice what has been culturally normal for them. Also, for black women who have more recently immigrated to the UK, breastfeeding they feel is a deep part of their mothering and how they interact with their babies/children.*
>
> *We must not forget that even if there is a strong desire or common cultural practice to breastfeed, there are still challenges that women face. Black women in the UK are often overlooked for breastfeeding support, because there is an assumption that black women know how to breastfeed. Though the statistics may show that black women are more likely to breastfeed, we need to look further into what this actually means.*
>
> *Many in the black community introduce formula top-ups or solids as early as 2–4 months, based on the belief that breastmilk is not a complete food for babies. There are black women who feel excluded from breastfeeding spaces, because often they don't feel represented in the support or the leadership. Therefore their stories, cultures and communities are not taken into account when helping women to meet their breastfeeding goals and, more widely, when trying to*

normalise breastfeeding and increase breastfeeding rates across the country. In my experience as a postnatal doula, black women want to breastfeed just as much as anyone else. Therefore, if we are to normalise breastfeeding and exclusive breastfeeding, black women must be included in the narrative and supported to breastfeed.

Looking further afield, you can see countless examples of the meaning breastfeeding can be given within communities around the world. As we will see in Chapter 6, in many parts of the UK breastfeeding rates are so low that formula is completely normalised and accepted as the 'normal and expected' thing to do.[12] However, in other countries the reverse is seen and women living in those countries, or who have come to live in the UK, can feel a need to breastfeed as it is part of what is expected of them – and they expect of themselves.

In these countries, breastfeeding (and thus those who breastfeed) is genuinely valued, embedded in societal norms that see motherhood as something precious and to be expected. This could be an entire book in its own right, and of course these attitudes and views cannot be generalised directly to women across countries. But it is interesting to consider how breastfeeding can be so tightly embedded in cultural identity. To explore this more deeply I spoke to Pamela Morrison, who lived in Africa (including in Kenya, Uganda and Tanzania) for 45 years, supporting women for over 13 years as a lactation consultant in Zimbabwe.

Children are highly valued in African societies and, by extension, so are their mothers. Women's status in society is elevated by being married, and by having children. As Claire Niala describes in Why African Babies Don't Cry, *in many societies a woman without a child is considered incomplete* and motherhood is a celebrated part of prominent women's credentials. And breastfeeding is an integral part of motherhood. It is not only seen as normal, and known to be a pillar of child survival – a way of keeping babies well nourished, healthy and happy – but there are other cultural and traditional beliefs associated with breastfeeding.

In many traditional African societies and certainly those in eastern, central and southern Africa, a breastfeeding baby is a visible sign to the rest of the community that his mother is a faithful wife and a good woman; one reason why you see babies being breastfed outside shops, on street corners, in banks, in public buildings and anywhere that women congregate. A baby who cannot or will not breastfeed, identifies his mother as having been unfaithful to her husband, the baby's father. Thus there is extremely high motivation to initiate breastfeeding as soon as possible after birth and to maintain breastfeeding well into the second or third years of life.

As an IBCLC in Harare, Zimbabwe, I worked with mothers and babies of all racial and ethnic groups. One case in particular brought home to me the crucial importance of an African baby being able to attach to the breast and breastfeed. I was asked to provide lactation help to a young African mother who had delivered a premature baby at a private clinic in the northern suburbs of Harare. The mother was distressed that her baby, born too early at about 30 weeks, was not breastfeeding. She was especially worried that her husband's family would think badly of her because the baby was not yet breastfeeding.

I was with her when the in-laws came to visit the new baby for the first time. Knowing their traditional beliefs, I explained carefully that he was not yet able to breastfeed because he was still too small and immature. But I confirmed that he was healthy and as time went on he would certainly be able

29

to. As expected he went on to breastfeed without problems. But it was not enough. Several months later her husband gave in to pressure from his family and divorced the mother. The shame attached to the baby's failure to breastfeed soon after birth was too great. On divorce in Zimbabwe often the father will take the children because they are deemed to be 'his'. But in this case, no one believed that the husband was the father of the baby, so the mother at least retained custody.

Alongside cultural beliefs and traditions, references to breastfeeding can be seen throughout historical and religious texts, meaning that breastfeeding can be an important part of following religious traditions as a mother. For example, in Hinduism, the primary sacred texts the Vedas (1800 BC) and other ancient Ayurvedic writings have many references to breastmilk, the breast and wet nursing, all in a context of bringing longevity. Breastmilk is life-giving – for example, when the god Shiva creates Parvati a baby boy out of her dress, he only comes to life when she puts him to her breast.[13]

Likewise, in Islam, there is specific reference in the Koran to breastfeeding for two years. Breastmilk is seen to belong to the baby – it is a gift from god and seen to be passing the mother's wealth onto the baby. Men are urged to support and enable their wives to breastfeed, and some Muslim women fear they will be punished if they do not breastfeed and fulfill this obligation.[14] As Maha Al Musa, birth mentor and founder of Embody Birth and Bellydance Birth, explains:

Breastfeeding signifies a symbiotic relationship of both nourishment and potent psychological harmonics between a mother and child. Personally it has informed my breastfeeding journey as a Palestinian Moslem woman with my own children to remember our matriarchal lineage that unites women in a circle of ancestral guidance. Our Islamic tradition encourages breastfeeding for two years and I deeply respect and honour the wisdom that has been a lifeline to mine and my children's historical sense of identity.

To be held in the belly of this womb with gratitude and connectedness has been one of enhancing my emotional and spiritual well-being. No one has the right to sever a mother and child from the well of this profound gift. I breastfed both my boys two years each and then my daughter, who was born at home when I was 46, was breastfed to natural term till she was 8.5 years and I was 54.5.

Finally, in Christianity, although there is no direct statement calling for babies to be breastfed, the Bible and religious texts are full of references to breastfeeding. Breastmilk and breastfeeding are associated with love, calm and security. Christian imagery often shows infants being nursed.[15] As Iyato Dunn reflected:

Breastfeeding is important to me for many reasons, many of which I didn't consciously think about when I started breastfeeding about five and half years ago. One of these reasons is my faith, the core of my very existence; permeating consciously and unconsciously through all I am and all I do.

In the darkness that enveloped the beginning of my first breastfeeding journey, my faith affirmed my biological instinct and overwhelming desire to feed my baby from myself. It fed my unending hope that I would somehow find a way to make enough breastmilk for my baby to eventually breastfeed him exclusively within the recommended 6 months of exclusive breastfeeding. It gave me the courage to let go of my psychological crutch of topping him up with expressed breastmilk about a week before I introduced solids into his diet, and instead trust that he could directly take all he needed from my breasts. It significantly contributed to my desire to learn about breastfeeding, and set myself up to physically and mentally make it work from the start, second time round.

You see, amidst my very difficult breastfeeding start, my belief that I am carefully and wonderfully made as the Psalmist stated in Psalm 139 took on a deeper meaning. I craved to know the breastfeeding aspect of this marvellousness within my created self for my child and I. I so wanted to walk in the fullness of the abundant life the book of John (10:10) states that Jesus came to give us. In my first major postpartum motherhood crisis, being able to continue sustaining my child fully from my breasts was part of the possible ways I felt I could know this fullness of life.

Whilst I'm not aware of a particular command to breastfeed in the Bible, I know from some of the biblical verses I've come across that breastfeeding is situated as a very valuable aspect of early motherhood, and it's a significant part of the imagery about the mother heart of God.

And so for me, persisting with breastfeeding against the odds, doing all I could to make it work when it all seemed bleak, committing to breastfeeding until my children don't want to anymore (despite years of nursing aversion and other challenges), and making sense of different aspects of breastfeeding, are all part of my faith journey. So, breastfeeding is another strand of my life through which I'm knowing God and making Him known; and I'm looking forward to doing a Bible study about breastfeeding soon.

Yet despite all this depth and complexity of belief and feeling, women are increasingly told that formula milk is a comparable substitute for breastfeeding. And to argue otherwise judges them or is anti-feminist.[16] While formula may feed the baby, women's desire to have their bodies work does not go away because they can formula feed. Women's feeling that their body has let them down does not go away because they can formula feed. Women's desire to mother in the way they want does not go away because they can formula feed.

To move forward we must invest in mothers. We may have breastfeeding promotion messages, but the support available for mothers is still lacking. Public health bodies are raising expectations, but failing to support and protect breastfeeding, or to provide answers if women cannot.[12] No wonder so much grief, hurt and anger abounds. We must stop telling women that their hopes and dreams when it comes to breastfeeding their baby do not matter.

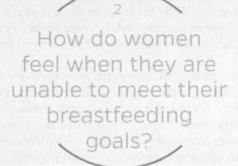

2

How do women feel when they are unable to meet their breastfeeding goals?

We've looked at why breastfeeding matters to women. But how do they feel when they can't? Some people are totally dismissive and think that it doesn't matter at all. The media offer just two options: women are 'bullied', or 'angry' about 'lactivists' pressurising them to breastfeed. Others seem to think the idea of breastfeeding being a 'goal' mothers might have is laughable or self-absorbed.

But what if we stop and listen to mothers? Few seem to get their voices properly heard. Women are misrepresented in stories designed to grab media headlines, or articles written with a particular agenda, presenting just one side of the story.

If you dig into the research literature on how women feel when they haven't been able to breastfeed, you can start to paint a much more detailed picture of how women feel. There are articles that talk about sadness and grief,[1] guilt and shame[2] and anxiety about harm to their baby.[3] Others talk about anger, perceived judgement and being made to feel inadequate.[4] But somehow the depth and breadth of these emotions doesn't quite come across. We have the outlines of the picture, but not the detail and colour.

I asked mothers '*How do you feel when you think back about your breastfeeding experience? What emotions do you feel?*' It was a simple question, but I did not get simple responses. Alongside the guilt and sadness I expected, was a full thesaurus of terms describing grief. Women didn't just feel sad – they felt robbed, bereft and defeated. Broken and traumatised. Devastated and exhausted. They talked about anger at everything letting them down: professionals, the system and their bodies. Their vulnerability was clear, with feelings of inadequacy, failure and helplessness. And at the heart of this was the loss. The grief. The trauma. To pick just one quote to sum this up, one woman described the all-encompassing physical nature of her grief:

> *It was a loss. A genuine loss to me that I felt physically through every part of my body. I mourned it like I would mourn somebody dying. I felt like somebody close to me had gone and I couldn't get them back. My whole body ached and I cried daily like I have never cried before. I genuinely have rarely known such sadness and it was such a shock to feel that way.*

I read every single story that women sent me. With over 2,000 stories, the process of reading through and understanding their words took over two years. The strength of their emotion was immediately obvious after the first few stories. It wasn't just about feeling a bit sad or guilty or annoyed when people talked about breastfeeding, it was so much more. Even many years after women had stopped breastfeeding the emotions were still there. For some, they had faded over time, but for others the mere mention of breastfeeding brought those emotions that were bubbling under the surface back to life.

These women's feeling could fill a whole book, but let's highlight just some of the key themes of the research here.

1. Feeling emotionally destroyed

The strength of that phrase really resonates doesn't it? It's not just feeling a bit sad or miserable, wishing things could be a bit different. Women feel genuinely bereft. As one mother explained:

I was completely emotionally destroyed by the experience. I spent months in a very black hole. I always saw myself as a breastfeeding mother and wanted to do it for so many reasons but I barely produced any milk. I was so shocked by that for a long time. How dare my body let me down like that? Did it not realise how important this was to me?

Others described the feeling of being crushed or broken by their experience. Whatever the word that was used, it is clear that this emotion is more than simply feeling a bit 'sad'.

Breastfeeding was really important to me. But on day 4 the hospital gave my baby formula. That just crushed me. On that day I felt they were taking my baby away from me. I felt sad when they said I had not enough milk, I felt like I myself was not good enough. I worked hard on pumping and taking care of my baby, I felt crushed.

For some these feelings turned to depression and dread, with a lasting feeling of misery attached to feeding. Feeding, and how they felt about it, took over their lives.

At the time I felt really depressed. It almost made me resent my baby that he wouldn't do the thing everyone was telling me should come naturally and be easy. I began to dread feeding him and in between feeds I would spend my whole time worrying about the next feed so wasn't bonding with my baby at all.

2. Feeling angry and shocked

Alongside feeling crushed, women described a strong sense of injustice about not being able to breastfeed for as long as they wanted. Women felt angry at themselves, their bodies and others – others who should have supported them, or others who they felt had an easy time breastfeeding or talked about it positively. The anger was deep and strong, with a sense of sheer unfairness about the whole situation. As one woman explained:

> [I felt] angry, really really angry and very sad. I refuse to feel guilty as I truly did everything I could at the time, but was undermined and didn't have the mental strength to believe in my body's ability to nourish my baby.

Shock was another core component of women's feelings, particularly among those who expected they would be able to breastfeed. Women talked about how they were rarely told that difficulties could arise, with education focusing on how to breastfeed and why it was a good idea. This shock was closely tied to anger – anger that they had been left feeling like this.

> It took me a long time to realise I wasn't going to be able to breastfeed him. I think I was genuinely in shock. I'd never considered any other option, never considered this would happen to me. Why hadn't anybody warned me?

3. Feeling like a failure

Failure was at the heart of many women's accounts. Failure to nourish their baby, as a mother and as a woman. Their stories showed just how important it is that we change this narrative, so that women stop shouldering and absorbing so much pain and realise that often they have been set up to fail. One woman wrote:

At the time, I felt like a failure and that I was letting my tiny baby down. I felt like everyone else had been able to do it but me. I felt very weak.

Although women's stories were full of examples of being let down by others, when they couldn't continue to breastfeed *they* were the ones who felt guilty, rather than realising that the blame lay elsewhere. As one woman recounted:

At first I was devastated and I felt horribly guilty. I thought I was failing my son, especially after we were readmitted to hospital as his weight loss was too high and he was basically starving. I felt under enormous pressure, not helped by the fact the hospital let me have a free meal because I was breastfeeding, and wouldn't if I wasn't. All health professionals seemed to put me breastfeeding above my own mental wellbeing, although this wasn't helped by the fact I saw three different midwives in the first five days after I gave birth who all had slightly different opinions. It took me a long time to not feel I had failed and to not feel so guilty.

4. Feeling guilty and ashamed

Feelings of shame and guilt permeated women's responses. How are we in a situation where women experiencing all of these difficulties end up blaming themselves? Women are being encouraged to breastfeed but then let down at every step, leaving them wracked with guilt. And many feel they are alone in this, not realising the sheer scale of the issue. They believe that they are a failure, and that they are the only ones to fail.

At the time, I felt very guilty that I could not breastfeed my son. I had many friends and family telling me that I wasn't trying hard enough, or that what I was experiencing was normal and I needed to push through the situation. I cried for hours and hours over this situation – I felt I must not be a strong enough person and questioned my ability to be a mother if 'everyone else' experienced the same thing and was able to continue breastfeeding – why couldn't I?

5. Feeling let down

Many women expressed frustration at the way in which they had been failed by others. Many had an issue where their baby had a health complication, or they were in considerable pain, or not producing sufficient milk, but could not find the support they needed. Things like tongue tie were missed, or women were told over and over that there was no problem and it was all in their head.

I also felt very frustrated with health professionals. I wanted to run away and leave my child, which was when I decided to stop trying to breastfeed. Eight months on I don't feel as upset about it now, just disappointed we were unable to do it. I still feel annoyed by what seems like constant breastfeeding campaigns when there was such poor practical support available for someone who really wanted to breastfeed.

Others were frustrated at the lack of treatment or diagnosis when something did go wrong. They expected, rightfully given how breastfeeding had been promoted to them as important, that if something was not right, there would be tests and support in place. Often there was no support and they were left with no answers.

At the time, I felt I had no support at all throughout my breastfeeding journey. I was so upset that the decision to stop breastfeeding was taken from me. I look back on it being a negative experience when it shouldn't have been. My baby latched from day 1 and I never experienced any pain until the abscess developed and I still don't understand why it did, I've been given no answers. I'm left with a physical scar on my breast, but the emotional scar remains – the experience of being in hospital where I felt the surgical staff didn't care or understand my emotional wellbeing.

6. Feeling envious of those who can

Others spoke of feelings of envy and jealousy, brought about when they saw others breastfeeding, particularly if they felt they were making it look simple and easy. This was often closely tied to how they felt about themselves as mothers, worrying that they had lost a bond with their baby that they felt others so effortlessly had or worrying that they were not doing the 'best' for their baby, when in the circumstances they really were.

I felt absolutely hopeless like I couldn't look after my own baby and that surely she didn't really need me if I couldn't feed her. It's not as strong now but I still feel gutted when I see other mums breastfeeding and I get out a bottle. It makes me tear up, as I so desperately wanted to do what was best for my baby but she was not putting on enough weight and I was put under a lot of pressure to give her formula.

7. Feeling lasting regret

Finally, women spoke of the regret they felt. Sometimes this feeling was there all along, but in other cases it replaced the anger and grief when they started to burn out. Notably women regretted not being able to breastfeed, but they also regretted how they were treated, with some regretting the context in which they had been a mother.

I feel regret. Let down by family. Let down by society for the perception that 'fed is best', that a baby should sleep, be content, be chubby, and if they are not then it is the fault of the breastfeeding.

I feel utterly failed by the NHS. I feel angry about the crappy society I was born into where women have been robbed of breastfeeding knowledge by formula companies. Initially, I grieved. I now feel regret every day.

The scale of the impact

What was also clear from my research was that for many women, their experience of breastfeeding had an impact in other areas of their lives. It started to affect how they felt about themselves as a mother, believing that if they were unable to breastfeed then in some way they were not caring for their baby 'properly', or were letting them down. Some felt that this way of mothering, without breastfeeding, was not what they envisaged mothering would be like.

Everyone around me breastfed – my aunts, my sisters, my cousins. When I was growing up someone was always breastfeeding. We were a big, close family and breastfeeding was normal to us. Certainly back in our home country in Ghana, absolutely everyone breastfed, it's just what you did as a mother. It was used all the time to help calm babies down or get them to sleep. Whenever a baby so much as whimpered someone in my family would say to feed that baby! To me it was how you cared for a baby, so when I couldn't do it I didn't know what to do. Even though the doctor said there was something wrong with my hormones and I would never make milk for my baby I don't think my family believed him and thought there was something wrong with me instead. I felt I was not a good mother and worry why I was made this way.

Some talked about how they felt everyone else was able to

breastfeed but they could not, adding to their feelings of failure as a mother. It was sadly all too common for mothers to feel that their baby was rejecting them, and somehow did not want, love or need them because they could not breastfeed.

I feel extremely guilty at my inability to feed my baby, especially because I had enough milk and she latched well, she just seemed to reject breastfeeding. At the time I felt as though my baby didn't love me. I no longer feel that way, but I'm desperately sad that I couldn't feed her myself.

Others talked about avoiding friendships because they could not breastfeed. Women really struggled to be around other breastfeeding women, especially those who they perceived as smug or who were having easy experiences. They knew that this was impacting on their friendships, but the strength of their emotion and grief overpowered this.

My best friend had a baby and it was so difficult to go see her. I am utterly ashamed that I did what I could to avoid her when she was breastfeeding, but now she's stopped I see her far more. I wish I had told her why but I couldn't and I worry our friendship will always be that little bit damaged because of how I feel.

Many women talked about how their emotions became so strong that they needed to be referred to a psychologist for support, or started taking antidepressants specifically because their experience of breastfeeding was so dreadful.

Horrible. Failure, sadness, disappointment. At the time of breastfeeding it was so bad my GP referred me to a psychologist for concerns about my mental health.

Who do women blame?

Every time I read about 'breastfeeding failure' in the media, what I find heartbreaking is the inevitable story at the centre of many women's experiences. It usually goes like this:

1. Woman really wants to breastfeed
2. Woman does not get the support she needs
3. Woman ends up blaming herself

As a society we are really quite good at getting women to feel guilty and blame themselves for stuff, aren't we? Everything is women's fault. Go right back to the garden of Eden and Eve and her tempting apple. Seriously, this is a societal problem. Women get layer and layer of guilt and responsibility and blame heaped on them every single day, almost from the moment they are born.

And breastfeeding it seems is no different. When I asked women who they felt was responsible for them feeling the emotions that they did, I had a wide range of responses, but the most common was sadly, and predictably, that a woman blamed herself.

It's all directed at myself. It's all me. I failed myself and her.

Some directed blame specifically at their body, feeling it had let them down and was broken. This is particularly distressing since we know that there is a wide gulf between how many women would never be able to physiologically breastfeed (a low percentage) and the number of women who end up stopping breastfeeding because of what happened to them – a lack of expert professional support, poor medical advice, a traumatic birth, myths about milk sufficiency and so on. This is further exacerbated by the lack of medical answers to breastfeeding problems. Women are left to feel abnormal, alone and like there is something wrong with them.

I am so angry at my body for not working. I have always had a love/hate relationship with my breasts as they are large and attracted so much male attention. But now I hate them and feel like they let me down just when they should have been doing what they were really put there for.

Others blamed someone other than themselves, which in some cases was a positive step to recognising the truth of the situation, and in other circumstances became a lot more complex. Sometimes blame can be useful. If you can redirect and attribute the emotions you feel to an external cause, particularly a justifiable one such as a lack of professional support, then feelings of guilt and failure can ease.[5] Many women were in this situation, blaming a lack of professional support. On one level this proved useful – they were recognising the issue and correctly attributing the blame. But the sheer scale of the rage and sense of being let down just further highlighted the awfulness of the situation in our society today. As one woman recalled:

I feel an absolute rage and fury that the GP told me I could not breastfeed and take the antidepressants I so desperately needed. Looking back I now know I could have. How dare he?

Some responses in particular showed an awareness of what is really going on in the world of breastfeeding – a lack of societal understanding, a lack of investment and commercial interests at play.

I feel fury that there is not enough support or money for breastfeeding, while formula companies get away with pushing their products and twisting facts.

This type of blame often led to positive outcomes – women

deciding to train as breastfeeding supporters, or fight the formula industry because they could see just how desperately other women need these barriers removing in the future.

Blame can become more problematic, however, if it falls on those close to you, causing damage to a relationship or family bonds, regardless of whether the blame is fairly attributed.[5] Many women felt this way. They blamed their partner for not helping – perhaps a justifiable blame to some extent (although the partner may well be caught in the wider societal issue of not knowing how to support a breastfeeding mother), but one that can be very damaging to a relationship.

I feel my husband should have supported me better. If I'd had his support then I wouldn't feel like this.

Others felt huge anger towards those they felt were promoting breastfeeding, feeling that whenever anyone talked about how they enjoyed breastfeeding, or encouraged others to breastfeed, that this was a direct attack on those who could not – making them feel guilty. This is of course something we see every day in the media, and which is deliberately stirred up.

I feel anger towards people who talk about breastfeeding because they know they are making people feel lesser parents.

There were also some desperately sad stories. Several women talked about how they felt blame and resentment towards their baby for not being able to breastfeed. Almost universally these statements were followed by the proviso that these feelings made them feel even worse.

I hate myself for it but I hated my baby. Why couldn't she do it like the other babies?

Why is breastfeeding grief so strong?

What is it about breastfeeding that brings such strong and lasting feelings, compared to other areas of parenting? I asked women whether they felt that breastfeeding grief was stronger compared to other areas where they had not been able to mother in the way they wanted, and why they thought that was. Many agreed that yes, on reflection, their grief was much stronger, and gave a number of reasons why they thought this was the case:

1. Its physiological nature
Feeding is so fundamental. If you can't get that right you feel like a failure.

2. The timing
Feeding your baby is the ultimate first guilt you feel as a parent.

3. Expectation
As a middle-aged, middle-class woman, the expectation was that I would breastfeed.

4. Lack of choice
In many other areas, not following suggested advice to the letter has been my choice. With regards breastfeeding, the choice was taken out of my hands making me helpless.

5. Tied to identity
It is seen as natural and you think if you can't do it then you are not and cannot be a good mother.

6. Desire
Yes, because breastfeeding was a thing I really really always wanted to do.

7. Omnipresence
Because it is so integral to that first six months especially, where feeding is everything, it's a pretty major area.

8. Others' reactions
It's the judgement. Like being at school and failing a test displeasing the teacher. Your child becomes someone else's property, you feel judged.

It is clear that we – as in society – have a major problem. Yes, we need to increase breastfeeding rates, because we have some of the lowest rates in the world.[6] But as a consequence of this we also have a maternal mental health crisis on our hands, because often attempts to promote breastfeeding fail to enable women to do so. It is not right that so many women are feeling this way, both because they are so badly let down by a lack of breastfeeding support, and because in a society that doesn't understand or value breastfeeding they are left blaming themselves. Women do not fail at breastfeeding – they are failed by a society that does not support them. And this is what we are going to change.

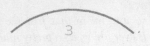
Breastfeeding, stopping breastfeeding and the risk of post-natal depression

The emotions described in the previous chapter are completely normal reactions to not being able to breastfeed for as long as you wanted to. Completely normal. But in the UK we're often not very good at dealing with difficult emotions. People feel awkward. They want to play your emotions down. They want you to get better quickly. Or they may simply dismiss the idea that things bothered you in the first place.

This seems to be especially true of grief attached to being a woman. Women's bodies and emotions are just a bit too complicated and messy for our society. And that's before we even get started on the discomfort we feel when women are angry, especially when it is anger directed at the patriarchal system that causes the things that make us angry.[1]

Grief is an utterly normal reaction to loss,[2] and we should probably all spend more time grieving when we lose things that are important to us rather than trying to push those emotions away. Many women identified their feelings as being a grief reaction, talking about the loss that they felt.

Feeling down, miserable or low about not being able to breastfeed is a normal part of a grief reaction.

> *It really did feel like a loss. I was mourning what should have been and the bonding experience I had been promised.*

As a society we should recognise this grief for what it is, and support and encourage women to be able to grieve that loss. As humans, sadness is something we need to feel and process, and it is a normal response to negative things happening in our lives. This is not to say it isn't completely awful when you're in the depths of it, but it does show you are having a healthy reaction to a negative thing.

> *It wasn't until I gave myself chance to properly grieve what had happened that I felt better.*

However, as we will see, it also helps if everyone around you recognises that a) you are sad, and b) this is an important loss to you. Ideally they will then support you through it rather than simply ignoring you or dismissing your feelings, as so often happens when it comes to breastfeeding.

But what about when you feel that sadness and it doesn't go away? When does normal grieving become something more complicated, or become a major contributor to or component of a more complex mental health issue? Unfortunately, breastfeeding experiences and postnatal depression can be closely tied together.[3] Mothers who plan to breastfeed but are not able to,[4] or who experience pain or difficulty that leads them to stop breastfeeding,[5] are more likely to experience postnatal depression. When breastfeeding goes well, a woman's risk of postnatal depression is lower, but when it doesn't go so well, her risk increases. There are so many reasons why these two things go hand in hand.

Breastfeeding helps protect good mental health

Let's start with the good bit. When breastfeeding goes well it can help women in many ways. As a group, women who are enjoying breastfeeding have lower stress and higher happiness levels than mothers who are bottle-feeding[3] (the key words in that sentence being 'when breastfeeding is going well').

There are both physiological and psychological reasons for this. Physiologically, the hormones of breastfeeding, particularly oxytocin, help you feel calmer and happier and help with bonding. Breastfeeding can help both mother and baby get more sleep.[6] At night, breastmilk contains melatonin, which helps a baby get to sleep (or back to sleep).[7] Higher prolactin levels can also help increase maternal slow wave and deeper sleep.[8] And it's also simpler to breastfeed a baby who has woken back to sleep. This might explain why research has shown that overall breastfeeding mothers report that they feel more awake and energetic, and physically healthier, than bottle-feeding mothers.[9]

There is also a fascinating body of research showing that breastfeeding appears to have a calming effect on the physical impact of stress on the body. More and more research is showing that depression and inflammation in the body caused by stress hormones are linked. Lots of things about early motherhood increase stress and inflammation – a lack of sleep, exhaustion and pain being just a few. But it appears that breastfeeding reduces that inflammation, in part by reducing the stress hormone response, which in turn reduces the risk of postnatal depression.[10]

Breastfeeding also seems to help a new mother's immune system if she is feeling stressed. Stress is associated with lower immune function. In one study of new mothers, stress and depression was associated with lower immune function, but only in mothers who were bottle-feeding. Mothers who were stressed but breastfeeding did not experience lowered immune function. A well-functioning immune system helps reduce your risk of getting sick and more stressed.[11]

And then there is the psychological side. As described earlier, in women who want to breastfeed, breastfeeding, if it is going well, is associated with all sorts of positive emotions, from feelings of pride and achievement through to spiritual calm and physical and psychological healing.[12] This experience in itself can boost a mother's wellbeing.

But when women can't breastfeed, they lose all these things. They lose the physical protection of breastfeeding hormones, and potentially gain a whole load of negative emotions, from grief to anger to loss, because their experience has not worked out as they hoped. Is it any wonder that they may feel depressed?

The experience of trying to breastfeed can increase depression

Mothers who care about breastfeeding enough to feel miserable when they stop, do not simply decide overnight that they don't want to breastfeed any more. Usually something significant, and often prolonged, leads to their decision to stop – whether that is insurmountable pain, a baby who just will not latch, a milk supply that will not increase, a health complication that is preventing breastfeeding or simply that she is overwhelmed by everything being too difficult.

It is unsurprising that it is these *reasons* for stopping breastfeeding that actually predict postnatal depression, rather than the stopping breastfeeding itself. A few years ago we did some research with mothers who had stopped breastfeeding in the first year and asked them why they had stopped breastfeeding. Specifically we asked them how strongly they agreed with eight core reasons for stopping. These were 'pain', 'difficulty', 'perceived inconvenience', 'body image', 'embarrassment', 'pressure from others', 'lack of professional support' and 'medical reasons'.[5]

We found two main things in that research:

1. How long a mother breastfed did not directly predict her risk of depression; rather, how ready she felt to stop predicted it. It didn't matter if her baby was 12 days old or 12 months old, if she hadn't been ready to stop her risk of depression was higher and vice versa.

2. If a mother stopped breastfeeding because of pain, physical difficulty or a lack of support, her risk of depression was higher. But if a mother stopped breastfeeding because she felt it was inconvenient and she *wanted* to move onto formula, her risk of depression fell. Again this shows that maternal desires and experiences really matter when it comes to infant feeding decisions.

It should come as no surprise that experiencing pain and physical difficulty during breastfeeding is linked to a higher risk of postnatal depression – and not simply because of losing the breastfeeding relationship. Women who had to stop for these reasons are likely to feel frustrated, angry and let down by a system that was meant to support them. But being in continual or regular pain, as a woman might well be if she has severe nipple damage or latch issues, is in itself depressing.[13] Babies who are difficult to feed are likely to feed very frequently, as they may well not be latching efficiently and not getting a lot of milk. Sleep deprivation is a strong predictor of depression,[14] exacerbated by the feeling that things will never get better and you're going to have to stop doing something that you really want to do.

The situation is made worse by the way our society treats new mothers. Women spend nine months growing brand new human beings, give birth to them, and then are on call 24/7, answering the needs of a tiny, helpless mammal (who doesn't want to be separated from her, wants to feed seemingly all the time and wants to sleep on her chest). In many other countries new mothers are cherished, with female relatives or friends taking on cooking and cleaning, and caring for the mother, so that she can rest and spend time getting to know her baby.[15]

For example, in Hindu culture a mother is expected to rest for 40 days after the birth. During this period she is excluded from housework in order to recover from the birth and care for her baby. Those around her provide her with regular, nourishing meals, alongside offering special foods that are believed in Hindu culture to increase the quantity and quality of her milk, including dried fish, dahl and aubergine.[16]

Compare this example to UK culture. How many mothers are caring for their newborn baby alone, miles away from family? How many have a partner who might be around for a week or so after the birth but is then back to work, feeling pressure to do well at their job to provide for their new family (or at the other extreme have used paternity leave to disappear and play golf)? How many visitors for new mothers actually care about her and her recovery, and how many are there to see the baby and expect to be waited on?

The problem is that the solution often offered to women – to stop breastfeeding – also increases their depression risk in a different way. It may remove the pain and it may, if they have a supportive partner, mean that they get more sleep. But stopping breastfeeding doesn't make all the tough things about caring for a baby in Western society suddenly go away – and it's all this other stuff that is likely making women feel so stressed. As one mother explained:

I was absolutely exhausted and overwhelmed with it all and a few people suggested I give up breastfeeding to get a break. I felt like a useless mother in so many other ways but the breastfeeding was the part I really loved and felt like I was doing a good job at. It helped me stop, escape and just be whilst I was feeding. It was all the other things I wanted to escape from and stopping breastfeeding wouldn't solve that.

Many mothers have to put up with the pressure from others to stop breastfeeding because they are depressed, with the implication that if they just stopped breastfeeding it would all be easier. Furthermore, some women find that if they say that breastfeeding is important to them and they want to continue, people get angry with them, saying that they are ignoring their advice and 'bringing it on themselves'. As one mother said in the research:

I hated my life and I hated myself. I thought I was a terrible, useless mother apart from breastfeeding, that was the one thing I was getting right. Why did everyone want to take that away from me?

Women are then left dealing with the loss of breastfeeding and anger that they were not supported. And we as a society seem surprised that they are depressed.

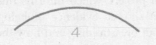

4

Can not being able to breastfeed cause psychological trauma?

We've talked about grief and we've talked about postnatal depression. But could it be, for some women, that their emotions around not being able to breastfeed are different? Might we actually be able to go as far as to say that women are experiencing clinical trauma because of their experiences?

It was an idle Tuesday afternoon when I first started to think about the concept of breastfeeding trauma seriously. I was procrastinating – sorry, I mean networking – on Twitter and reading a thread about the terrible ways in which women are let down when it comes to breastfeeding. I made a number of comments, but one in particular was noticed. I simply posted *'I'd go as far to say that these women are traumatised'*.

And almost immediately, up popped a middle-aged, white, male academic who informed me that *I could not* use that word when it came to breastfeeding women. I don't know about you, but the one thing guaranteed to push my buttons is being told I cannot do something. Especially by someone who I assume had never used his nipples to feed a baby. So I embarked on three years of research into the subject to prove him wrong.

That research project, which informs this book, explored whether women showed evidence of being traumatised in their stories about breastfeeding and how they feel about it. I can now confidently say that yes, some women really do show clinical signs of trauma due to their experiences. Of course, not every woman who can't breastfeed and feels negatively about it is 'traumatised'. But some are and the impact on them is clear.

What is trauma?

The concept of trauma, or post-traumatic stress disorder (PTSD), was first described in response to symptoms soldiers suffered on coming home from war. They had nightmares and flashbacks, startled easily and experienced a whole range of emotions including anger, sadness and self-blame.

Subsequently, clinical criteria were put in place to diagnose conditions like PTSD. These criteria typically focused on a serious, life-threatening event being central to any trauma experience. For example, the *Diagnostic and Statistical Manual Version Five* (*DSM V*) classifies different mental health issues according to a list of symptoms and experiences. The *DSM V* identifies a traumatising event as one in which:[1]

The person was exposed to: death, threatened death, actual or threatened serious injury, or actual or threatened sexual violence either through 1) direct exposure, 2) witnessing the trauma in person, 3) indirectly by learning that a close relative was exposed to the trauma, or 4) indirect exposure to adverse details of the event usually in the course of professional duties.

This definition of an event as traumatic is stark – it must involve either death itself, or a fear that you or someone else was going to die. It is far removed from the use of the word 'trauma' in everyday language. A similar diagnostic tool, the

International Classification of Diseases (ICD), version 10, is slightly broader, defining trauma as:[2]

> *A delayed or protracted response to a stressful event or situation (of either brief or long duration) of an exceptionally threatening or catastrophic nature, which is likely to cause pervasive distress in almost anyone.*

However, this definition of an event is still severe, suggesting a physical rather than emotional threat. So can breastfeeding ever fit these definitions?

I argue yes, for several reasons. Firstly, although in most cases no lasting physical damage will have occurred, might the body on one level perceive a loss? Breastfeeding is an instinctual part of the reproductive process. It is what mammals naturally do with their baby once it is born. Again, this is not to be confused with an imperative – that a mother *should* do something – but hormonally, physiologically, the female body produces milk after birth (unless something is wrong). All this is primitive and automatic. It does not involve conscious, human-level thinking and rationalising. Thus, if the baby is not put to the breast, the primitive part of a woman's body and brain may think that something is very wrong with her baby, or even that her baby has died.

This way of thinking may seem too 'evolutionary' for some. Thinking about it in another way, however, many women who have not been able to breastfeed have experienced significant physical trauma or injury along the way. A difficult birth (physically or emotionally), which we now recognise can lead to trauma,[3] is often bound up with breastfeeding difficulties – both from a physiological and hormonal point of view, and because a woman may feel a loss of confidence in her body's ability.[4] Babies who are sick at birth are more likely to end up in special care, which is a known trigger or exacerbator of birth trauma –

and again, a known risk for breastfeeding complications.[5]

Focusing on breastfeeding complications alone, if a mother is not producing enough milk and not getting the medical input she needs, and her baby is losing weight rapidly, perhaps becoming dehydrated or worse – is that not traumatic? Being told your baby isn't getting enough milk, feeling an urgency and pressure to produce more, and worrying about their health – is that not traumatic? Or for some, knowing your baby will need formula but worrying about the impact on their health – is that not traumatic?

And that's before we look at injury – and I say that making no light of it – the real injury some mothers end up with after not receiving the expert guidance they need. Abscesses, bleeding nipples, nipples that are half detached and raw, and continuing to put the baby to the breast over and over every two hours or more often[6] – how on earth is that not trauma?!

Finally, a number of the risk factors for trauma are also risk factors for having a difficult breastfeeding experience. These include: a sick baby, existing maternal mental health issues, pain, and a lack of support.[7]

It seems clear that some women will therefore meet that first criterion of trauma. Furthermore, our understanding of what constitutes trauma, outside of strict definitions and diagnosis, is becoming much broader. These days the focus is much more on a person's emotional experience rather than their physiological state, and a more holistic view is taken by those supporting people in the community who have experienced trauma, for example through local mental health support teams, rather than relying on the clinical definitions a psychiatrist might use.[7] The NHS is increasingly taking people's emotional experiences, such as their childhood, or stressful ongoing events at work or in relationships, as indicative of trauma.[8]

Here are some wider definitions of trauma. Do you think

they are a fitting description of how some women feel when they cannot breastfeed?

- *Individual trauma results from an event, series of events, or set of circumstances that is experienced by an individual as physically or emotionally harmful or life-threatening and that has lasting adverse effects on the individual's functioning and mental, physical, social, emotional, or spiritual well-being.*[9]
- *The individual's ability to integrate his/her emotional experience is overwhelmed.*[10]
- *Psychologically, the bottom line of trauma is overwhelming emotion and a feeling of utter helplessness.*[11]

The idea that emotional experience and subjective interpretation is at the heart of determining whether an event is traumatic or not is recognised as being central to birth trauma, which has a lot of similarities with how some women feel about their feeding experiences. Birth trauma is not defined by a checklist of procedures and interventions that are considered traumatic, but involves the realisation that how a woman felt (or was made to feel) during her birth can lead to lasting trauma.[9] This can include:

- Feeling out of control
- Feeling helpless
- Feeling scared
- Feeling like no one is supporting you
- Feeling abandoned
- Feeling ignored
- Worrying about your baby's health and safety
- Blaming yourself
- Being made to feel as if you don't matter
- Being told it doesn't matter

Ultimately, it has been recognised that how safe or unsafe a woman feels during her birth – physically and emotionally – can be a trigger for birth trauma.[6] Again, thinking about the experiences many women have when they experience complications trying to breastfeed their baby – how many can be ticked off? All of them.

Why else might breastfeeding experiences lead to trauma?

Looking at the wider trauma literature, which describes those factors that increase the likelihood that someone will experience trauma, there are several pertinent factors that are present in many women's breastfeeding experiences.[9]

1. It's a difficult memory to escape

Some people with trauma manage to keep it out of their mind by avoiding traumatic reminders. If, for example, they experienced an air travel emergency, they might try to avoid planes, or if they experienced birth trauma, they might try to avoid the hospital in which they gave birth. This is not the recommended way to deal with a traumatic event, but shows that sometimes avoiding triggering situations is possible.

Now take feeding your baby. When you can't breastfeed, your baby still needs feeding. Every few hours you have to prepare a bottle of milk and give it to your baby. It's a visual reminder. Everywhere you go as a new mother, there are other new mothers feeding their babies. You go along to a baby group and there are women breastfeeding. The local coffee shop... women breastfeeding. Even on the tin of formula milk it tells you that breastfeeding is best for your baby. Reminder after reminder. Over and over all day long. Week in, week out. Is it any wonder that women don't have time to heal?

2. We blame ourselves for not being able to breastfeed

As we have seen, when women cannot breastfeed they often blame themselves. And this is a key feature in lasting trauma.[15]

Various models of trauma state that how we as individuals determine whether something is traumatic or not depends on how we explain it. If we think that a traumatic event was a freak, one-off, completely random thing that is unlikely to happen again, then we are less likely to be traumatised. If, however, we think we are responsible for it, that we could have avoided it, and that it is ultimately down to us… then this can embed a trauma more deeply.

As we saw in the previous chapter, many women hold themselves responsible for not being able to breastfeed. And they tie that trauma so closely to themselves because breastfeeding was part of their vision of motherhood, part of their identity. So they feel, subconsciously at least, that the trauma was their fault and reflects on them as a mother.

3. So many people do not take breastfeeding seriously

Despite messages encouraging women to breastfeed, many women find that once their baby is here, and they are struggling, the solution is to give a bottle. And they are told it doesn't matter. And that they should be happy and grateful that their baby is alive and fed.

The problem with this attitude, as we will see in more detail later, is that although some might be comforted by it, many who care deeply about breastfeeding are ultimately made to feel much worse. They feel as if their wishes, desires and identity are being dismissed. Of course, everyone wants a healthy, fed baby, but that isn't the only thing that matters, nor should it ever have to be an either/or situation. It is perfectly possible to be grateful that your baby is fed, and simultaneously broken by the fact you could not breastfeed.

This is all scarily reflective of the messages women receive around birth and trauma. In her book *Why Birth Trauma Matters*, also in this series, Dr Emma Svanberg talks about how trauma around childbirth is often ignored or dismissed. She gives the example of a car crash. If you had a car crash and were in hospital everybody would be focused on you – expecting you to be physically and emotionally traumatised by the experience and validating and confirming your experience as traumatic. But when a woman has a traumatic birth, it's as if everyone forgets about her and instead just keeps asking if her car was alright. If your car survived the crash ('all that matters is a healthy baby'), then that's the main thing, right? Women feel that they are mistaken or wrong to find the experience traumatic, and the same applies to breastfeeding.[16]

What are the symptoms of being traumatised?

There is increasing recognition that perhaps we should spend less time focusing on what *happened* when determining whether someone is traumatised, and instead look at their *symptoms*.[10] Trauma can mean different things to different people.

Take divorce for example. Is that stressful? How stressful? Older theories of stress were based on the idea that divorce, or death, or a house move were all stressful, and people were given a 'score' for each stressful event they experienced. Then we realised that stress was far more subjective than that. Some people will be broken by a divorce. Others will throw a party to celebrate.

It seems clear that we should not only be asking whether someone has experienced an objectively traumatic event, but also considering their reaction to events. If you look at the checklists in the *DSM V* and *ICD 10* for what constitutes trauma, many of the points are based on how individuals then react to a traumatic event. For example, in the *DSM V* there is a list of different criteria and symptoms that are used to determine whether symptoms of trauma are being experienced:[1]

1. Intrusion symptoms

The first of these are known as 'intrusion symptoms' or, in other words, does the individual become overwhelmed by thoughts and reminders of the event, despite not wanting to think about it? This includes things like intrusive thoughts (recurrent, involuntary and intrusive memories), nightmares, dissociative reactions (e.g. flashbacks), intense or prolonged distress after exposure to traumatic reminders, and marked physiologic reactivity (physical symptoms) after exposure to trauma-related stimuli. As you might expect, many mothers' stories included symptoms that met this criteria. Mothers talked about being 'triggered' by seeing breastfeeding, or hearing others' stories. Both positive and negative connotations of breastfeeding could trigger these emotions, which were involuntary and vivid.

> *When I read articles that go on about how great breastfeeding is I'm right back in those dark days with him screaming for hours and hours a day.*

These could appear during the day in reaction to seeing or hearing about breastfeeding, or present as recurrent nightmares:

> *I have a regular dream where I'm back in hospital and trying to get support for my dehydrated baby and I can't. It goes on and on where I'm begging for help but no one can hear me and each time I fail to get help my baby shrinks a little more. I always wake up just before he disappears, dripping in sweat and my heart pounding.*

2. Avoidance

This describes the different ways in which a traumatised individual will avoid events that remind them of their trauma.

These include trauma-related thoughts or feelings, or trauma-related external reminders such as people or places. Again, as you would expect, avoidance behaviours were seen in many mothers' responses. Some reported avoiding anything breastfeeding related, blocking groups on Facebook or making sure they did not read articles about breastfeeding.

I can't read anything about breastfeeding or babies in general. It's too traumatic still. I am a bit better now but went through a phase where I even needed to avoid the baby aisle in the supermarket as it would trigger how I felt or put me on edge for the rest of the day without realising why.

Others felt completely out of control, trying to stop themselves from reading stories about breastfeeding but not able to. They knew it would hurt and trigger emotions, but kept going:

I have blocked lots of social media accounts and pages so they can't get to me but sometimes an article slips through and I'm compelled to read it. I always wish I hadn't but can't stop myself even though it can trigger terrible anxiety.

Some women reported that their attempts to avoid breastfeeding had actually changed their lives. Mothers would avoid baby groups that they once visited, or even stop seeing friends and family members who were breastfeeding new babies. Friendships were changed and even lost, because mothers were simply not able to be around breastfeeding.

I do everything I can to avoid one friend who is a real lactivist. She is lovely and would hate to know she hurts me but I can't bear to hear her talk about her struggles breastfeeding her two-year-old.

3. Negative alterations in cognitions and mood

This relates to negative thoughts or feelings that began or worsened after the trauma, such as shame, guilt, self-blame, feeling isolated or detached, or not being interested in pre-trauma activities. Obviously, in stories of women who feel negatively about not being able to breastfeed, you would expect most of them to have a tick in this box! Guilt was a core feature in many stories. What is important is to consider the depth and breadth of these emotions.

How do I feel? Everything. I am angry and sad and guilty all at once.

A common experience was for women to find that, despite feeling so negatively about their experience, their actual specific memories of it were quite blurred, seeming almost unreal at times.

I find it increasingly hard to remember that time. It's like my brain has blocked it out to stop me from hurting myself.

The strength of women's emotions was particularly strong here. Again, women were not a 'bit sad' or 'fed up', they used words like 'hate' and 'despise'. Blame was also a core feature – directed at themselves and others.

I hate myself and think I am not a good enough mother. Nothing anyone says or does can change the fact I failed.

I despise the GP who failed to diagnose my son's tongue tie. I really think it's all his fault and there should be consequences. I reported him but nothing has been done. Why is it fair I feel this way when he feels nothing?

This criterion also involves the idea of being uninterested in activities that you once enjoyed. Some women talked about this broadly – feeling a lack of interest or flatness at once-cherished activities. One woman explained, in a line I felt was one of the saddest in the whole study, that her experience of not being able to breastfeed had had a profound effect on her social connections and identity, as previously she had been well known in breastfeeding support circles.

I'm struggling as I was a big advocate in my community. I've been pretending I'm too busy with three children now but really it's because I can't bring myself to talk about breastfeeding and see other mothers who are able to.

Sadly this was not an isolated case; other women talked about how they became more and more distanced from their previous lives.

4. Alterations in arousal and reactivity
This relates to the physical symptoms an individual can experience as a direct consequence of trauma. Two of the following are needed for diagnosis: irritability or aggression, risky or destructive behaviour, hypervigilance, heightened startle reaction, difficulty concentrating, and difficulty sleeping.

Anger, irritability and destruction featured in women's stories. Often they knew what was happening. They could see themselves getting angrier, but couldn't stop it.

I have lost friendships over arguments with breastfeeding. I see red and can't help myself and find myself calling them awful things. I know it's because I'm hurting but I can't seem to stop myself pressing the destruct button and making things even worse than they already are.

Others reported feeling on edge, primed and ready to make sure they wouldn't encounter any information that made them feel negative.

I do everything I can to avoid breastfeeding to the point of excluding potentially great new friendships. I even do things like scan their social media to see if they post breastfeeding articles or belong to groups and if they do I hide them from my wall.

Many women talked about how, when they were in the grip of trauma, they found it really difficult to concentrate or sleep. Everything was affected, and although for some this was because they were playing their experiences over and over in their minds, others just felt agitated and restless, unable to relax.

I find myself getting preoccupied with babies and breastfeeding long after I read an article. It plays on my mind and goes round and round and I find it difficult to concentrate on what I should be doing so I try to avoid reading anything just in case.

How long have you felt this way?

Aside from these criteria, two further things need to be taken into consideration when thinking about whether or not an individual is traumatised. The first of these is duration, or in other words, how long the feelings have lasted. In the *DSM V* it suggests the symptoms must have lasted at least a month. This takes into account the fact that it is normal to feel all of the above in reaction to a traumatic event. It would perhaps be a sign that something was wrong if you experienced a deeply traumatic event and were absolutely fine afterwards. But it also recognises that if an individual is 'okay' then they will gradually start to get better over the next few weeks. If the trauma is to be more lasting, the symptoms will persist longer, even getting worse.

I asked mothers in the research how long they had been feeling this way. The youngest baby was three weeks old, and the mother's feelings were very recent and raw. However, the vast majority of mothers had a baby whom they had stopped breastfeeding at least a month ago, yet their feelings were still present.

The oldest baby in the study was 36 years old. Thirty-six years and the mother still felt the hurt and the guilt and the frustration at the system. She described how her emotions had eased over time, and changed, moving away from self-blame towards recognising she had been let down, and blaming that system that let her down. But it still hurt. And when she heard about other women experiencing breastfeeding difficulties it brought so much back to her of how she felt.

Women tell me stories like this all the time. Of babies who now have dodgy facial hair and mortgages, or even in one case, who had just retired. Breastfeeding grief and trauma last. Women hold it with them and carry it around, in a world that keeps on letting women down and telling them it doesn't matter.

Would you say it is interfering with your life?

The last criterion for trauma is that symptoms must create distress or functional impairment (getting in the way of an individual's usual social or occupational roles). This was common, with mothers explaining how their feelings impinged on their day-to-day activities. For some this was mild, such as blocking articles on social media, but for others it had a severe impact on their ability to maintain existing elements of their lives.

I try to avoid seeing friends who are particularly breastfeeding happy. I know it's not healthy to do this but it stops me getting upset and should only last a while. I think they know what I'm doing but they understand, although it doesn't seem to stop them talking about how wonderful they find breastfeeding.

Of particular concern was the number of women who recognised that their experience would make their return to work very difficult. Midwives, health visitors and GPs all talked about the anxiety they felt, worrying about how they would support women when they felt so badly let down themselves.

I'm a midwife and am dreading returning to work as how am I meant to support new mothers now?

Does a positive next breastfeeding experience help?

Before I collected the data, I had in my mind that perhaps if women went on to have another baby, and tried breastfeeding and it worked out for them, then this might help heal them. I'd heard stories from mothers who had a traumatic birth the first time around, but in the second birth had felt far more in control and had a positive birth experience. These mothers often said that they felt that the second birth helped heal the first birth. Their body worked. They felt cared for. Listened to. And empowered. This concept has also come up in previous research looking at birth trauma, although of course not all women will feel this way.[5]

I didn't directly ask women about their subsequent feeding experiences, but many women spoke about them. And I was shocked to see that for many the exact opposite seemed to be true. When women couldn't breastfeed their first baby, but went on to successfully breastfeed their second baby, it was as if all the trauma came pouring out. They realised that their body was capable and that the circumstances of their first baby were actually to blame. They realised just how badly they had been let down. And knowing that made them so angry and frustrated by their first experience that all those feelings of being let down came back twice as strong.

This is why I will never let some random man on Twitter tell everyone that a woman's experience of trying to breastfeed can never be considered traumatic.

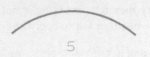

Why do so many women struggle to breastfeed?

I just always knew I was going to breastfeed. I didn't even bother looking at formula even for the occasional feed. But then he was born, and he just wouldn't latch. We tried everything, over and over but he just couldn't get it. I expressed for him at first, but my milk just never really came in fully and what milk I did have steadily dropped over the first few days until there just didn't seem any point any more. I was so upset that I couldn't breastfeed him but more than that somehow, I was shocked. I mean I was a middle-class, well-educated woman – the poster girl almost for breastfeeding. I didn't expect anything else to happen but breastfeeding. What went so wrong?

The story above is the story of countless women. Although the exact details may be different, the underlying structure is the same. They wanted to breastfeed, did everything they could to try and breastfeed, yet somehow they couldn't and this blindsided them. They certainly aren't alone. In the UK over 80% of women want to breastfeed their baby and do so at least for one feed. But then the rate plummets rapidly. Even by the end of the first week more than half of babies have received formula milk, with less than half breastfeeding *at all* by six weeks, and only a third having *any* breastmilk by six months. And that's before you even begin to consider exclusive breastfeeding. Just 1% of mothers reach six months of exclusive breastfeeding.[1]

The key point about these statistics for me is that they don't represent what women *want* to do. Research shows that out of those women stopping breastfeeding in the first six weeks, the vast majority – some research suggests up to 90% – were not ready to do so.[1] They are not stopping because they've had enough, or because they think something else will be easier, but because they feel they have to – that breastfeeding is insurmountable.

So what's going on? Is breastfeeding really so difficult that it simply doesn't work for hundreds of thousands of women every year? There are several things to think about here. First, there are many, many reasons why women are not able to breastfeed when they want to, including physiological, cultural and social reasons. Some women will have a health complication that prevents them from breastfeeding, but for many others, their complex experiences will lead them to a place where they are unable to breastfeed.

This is illustrated by the vast difference in breastfeeding rates around the world. While rates in the UK are among the lowest in the world, those in developing regions are much higher – almost universal at birth, with the vast majority of women continuing into the second year and beyond. However, rates can be high in developed regions too. In many Scandinavian countries, at least two-thirds of women are breastfeeding at six months, compared to a third in the UK. This goes to show that it cannot be purely physiological issues that are preventing women from breastfeeding – something complex is going on at the societal level that is directly or indirectly harming their ability to breastfeed.[2]

So why are so many women struggling? Let's break it down into those two broad reasons – the physiological reasons why some women will never be able to breastfeed (or do so exclusively), and the psychosocial reasons why women stop breastfeeding, often because they end up with too little milk.

Physiological factors that affect breastfeeding

We simply don't have an accurate estimate of how many women have a reason why they would never be able to breastfeed their baby, or would be advised not to. Complete lack of milk production (primary insufficient milk supply) is very rare – but it does happen. Other women will not make a full milk supply no matter what they try, or it will be very delayed, meaning their baby ends up needing to be formula fed in the early days. But it's important to remember that even when we say these circumstances are rare, we mean statistically, across a large population. In reality, if just 1% of women have a physiological problem, that is approximately 7,000 women each year when you consider that around 700,000 women give birth each year in the UK.

Primary insufficient milk supply

I barely produced any milk at all in the early days. When I tried to hand express just a few drops came out. This did increase but by day five my baby had lost a lot of weight and I was advised to give him some additional formula. I did everything I could to try to get to a stage where I was fully breastfeeding him. I fed him. Then I topped him up with formula. Then once he was settled I tried and tried to express to persuade my milk supply to increase but only ever got a very small amount out and was making myself really sore. It wasn't until I eventually saw a lactation consultant two weeks later that she said by looking at me she thought that perhaps I didn't have enough of the tissue needed to make enough milk. I searched online for this and it all made sense. My breasts just hadn't developed like most did. I guess I knew this but I thought it was just about how they looked rather than whether I could feed my baby or not. Why didn't anyone tell me?

Women who have insufficient glandular tissue (often called hypoplasia, or tubular breasts) can find it difficult to make a full milk supply for their baby no matter what their experience is after birth. This doesn't mean they won't produce any milk, but often they won't be able to exclusively breastfeed their baby. Women with this condition have breasts that typically lack fullness, the areola is often enlarged, and breasts are widely spaced and low. Often there is very little change in breast shape or size during pregnancy or after birth, but unless women are specifically looking out for this and realise it is a sign that something is wrong, it may be missed.[3]

If a woman has had a breast reduction this may also affect her milk supply, depending on exactly what surgery was performed. If lots of glandular tissue and ducts were removed, or her nipple and areola were removed and repositioned, this may mean less milk is produced. Any cuts near the areola can affect supply as the nerves that send a signal for milk to be produced and let down might be affected.[4] Conversely, breast implants are usually okay, especially if they are placed under the muscle wall and incisions are away from the nipple.[4]

Chronic health conditions

I'd been on thyroid replacement medication for ten years and my dose was tweaked in pregnancy. But no one thought to mention that my thyroid condition might affect my milk supply. I actually asked my GP when my baby was six weeks old whether he thought my thyroid issues were leading to lower milk supply and he dismissed it saying my thyroid was just fine and I was just a tired, emotional new mother. He suggested I let my husband feed the baby a bottle so I could get some sleep and that would sort it all out. It didn't and it took me pushing repeatedly for more tests to show my thyroid wasn't under control at all. By the time I got it sorted I had stopped breastfeeding as the sheer exhaustion meant I couldn't carry on. I'm so angry at him as if someone had told me in pregnancy this could happen we would have been able to plan it better.

There are a number of chronic health issues which can affect milk supply, but again many women report that these are just not discussed with them before their baby is born.[5] As in the example above, an underactive thyroid can affect milk supply if it is not under control. Unfortunately the hormonal changes after birth and lack of sleep can mean thyroid levels are all over the place, affecting milk supply and leaving women feeling too exhausted to put up a fight for the care they deserve. Diabetes can also affect supply as insulin is involved in milk production, so if insulin levels are too low after birth, or not being managed correctly in the chaos of a new baby, milk can be delayed or low in volume. Finally, women with polycystic ovarian syndrome (PCOS) may find their supply is too high, or too low. Very few are told about this during pregnancy.

Illness
Some women find out that their baby has an illness that means they have to have a specialised formula and will never be able to tolerate breastmilk.[6] These disorders are very rare and include galactosaemia and phenylketonuria. Galactosaemia is diagnosed via the heel prick test babies have in the first week. It is a metabolic disorder in which not enough of the enzymes needed to break down and digest lactose and galactose in milk are produced. Babies with this condition will need a specialist

soy-based formula. Some babies with galactosaemia have a type called Duarte galactosaemia, which means they can produce limited amounts of the necessary enzymes and can receive some breastmilk alongside specialist formula. Similarly, babies with phenylketonuria cannot break down part of a protein in milk known as phenylalanine, so they again need specialised formula, although as breastmilk is naturally low in phenylalanine they can receive small amounts.

Sometimes mothers are ill with a disease that means they cannot give their baby their breastmilk because it will be transferred via the milk. These illnesses are fairly rare and include Ebola, untreated brucellosis and human T-cell lymphotrophic virus. HIV is another illness which presents a dilemma. Although in developing regions women with HIV are encouraged to continue exclusive breastfeeding, as HIV presents a lower overall risk than not breastfeeding, in developed regions women are often advised not to breastfeed, unless the baby is already infected with HIV.[7] However, the World Health Organization states that women should be counselled about the risks involved and enabled to make a decision that is right for their family. The risk of a baby contracting HIV through breastmilk if a mother is taking antiretroviral therapy (ART), her viral load is low and she is breastfeeding exclusively without cracked nipples or thrush, is almost negligible.

For some other illnesses, the virus or infection will not get into the breastmilk, but the mother may be contagious. This includes things like tuberculosis, varicella or active herpes lesions. However, expressed milk can be given to the baby and may help protect the baby if any contact has been made.[8]

Medications

Unfortunately I developed postnatal depression with my second daughter and after trying to ignore it for a few weeks I made an appointment with the GP. She said I was depressed and had to start taking care of myself and that meant taking antidepressants and unfortunately I couldn't breastfeed on those. I was absolutely gutted but took them and it wasn't until a few months later that someone told me I could have carried on taking them. I despise that GP. Not only did they not do much for me, but she took away the one thing that mattered to me and I felt I was really good at.

Unfortunately, being prescribed a medication is a common reason for women to be told they need to stop breastfeeding. Although some medications should not be taken during breastfeeding, such as lithium, chemotherapy and methotrexate for arthritis, the majority of medications are safe to take during breastfeeding as they either do not enter breastmilk or do so in very small amounts. Sometimes a different medication is needed, or a short break from breastfeeding is required, but there is usually an option which protects breastfeeding in the long term.[8]

However, our research with women who had contacted Drugs in Breastmilk (an information service run by the Breastfeeding Network for women to check the safety of medicines or medical procedures while breastfeeding) showed how common it is for women to be wrongly told that they must stop breastfeeding. Women are frequently told that they cannot breastfeed on common medications such as antidepressants, antihistamines, antibiotics and emergency contraception[9] when this is completely false.

So it is clear that some women will never be able to breastfeed. But where is the support for them? Few are made aware of these issues during pregnancy and have a plan put in place for support. Few are asked how they feel when they are then unable to breastfeed. Why are women who are struggling with milk supply and don't understand why, not given access to tests, experts and diagnoses? Too often they are told to give a bottle instead.

Psychological, social and cultural factors that affect breastfeeding

Unfortunately, many women who are not able to breastfeed have had their ability to do so damaged by the wider environment. Although they desperately want to breastfeed, factors such as a lack of professional support, critical friends and family, a lack of societal understanding around how breastfeeding works and pressures on women to get their life back or return to work can all make breastfeeding seem impossible. The messages and pressures women experience can have an impact physiologically – reducing milk supply and leading them eventually to stop breastfeeding. So what are these factors?

A lack of professional support

All the way through pregnancy women are told that breast is best for their baby. Are you going to try breastfeeding your baby? You know breastfeeding helps your baby stop getting sick, right? Are you going to give it a go?

And then the baby is born… and many women find themselves with no support.

Not being able to get the professional support they needed to breastfeed is central to many women's journeys to stopping breastfeeding. Before I go any further, I want to say that there are many excellent health professionals out there desperate to support new mothers. But government cuts to breastfeeding support services under the name of austerity have led to many women being unable to get through even the first few days. Midwives are rushed off their feet and unable to sit and take the time to support women with breastfeeding. Services in the community are stretched to breaking point or have been dismantled.[10]

Breastfeeding might be the most natural thing in the world, but that does not make it easy. In previous generations we wouldn't have needed the same level of formalised support to breastfeed that we do now. For a start we would have grown up seeing babies breastfed and knowing how it all worked. We would also have been having babies as part of communities in which everyone had breastfed and knew how to help. Today, most people's dominant experience is of bottle-feeding, and no matter how much they want to help, they can't (more on this later). Instead, women need the support of trained, skilled professionals who can help them with positioning and attachment, tell them what is normal, and help them with any problems that crop up.

What happens when women encounter this lack of support?

It was like someone sticking a knife in me. The midwife in the hospital told me my latch was fine but I used to have to bite down on a pillow and scream at the start of each feed. The only option for support was to go to the baby clinic but I just couldn't face it. I stopped and things eventually healed but I hated myself for being so weak. I felt I should have just toughened up a bit and got through it and often wonder now whether that physical pain would be preferable to the regret I feel now.

If the baby does not latch properly to the breast, they get less milk, and their mother ends up in pain. And not just a bit of soreness – nipple half-hanging-off type pain. Obviously, when you're in that amount of pain you might try and delay feeding. Or give a bottle to give yourself a break. But the less a baby feeds, the fewer signals are given for more milk to be produced, and the more a woman's milk supply drops. That's if she can bear feeding at all. Pain is not just painful… it's exhausting, demoralising and depressing.[11]

It is unsurprising that experiencing pain is one of the most common reasons for stopping breastfeeding. What's rage-inducing is that many women experiencing such pain would find relief with the right support. They need the midwife to have the time to sit with them. They need that one-to-one home-visiting health service. They need that peer support group to drop into where someone can spot that things aren't right and refer them to the local specialist infant feeding midwife. Maybe their pain is more complex and they need a lactation consultant.

A lack of investment in support at all levels means that women don't get what they need. The midwife is caring for too many women, all of whom need her. The health visitor has been forced to set up clinic-only appointments, which are always rammed. The peer support group has had their funding cut and the specialist infant feeding supporter lost her job. No one mentioned the lactation consultant.

Our research shows that when women stop breastfeeding because they are in pain or having practical difficulties, their risk of postnatal depression soars.[12] What's so infuriating is that we know what the solution is! When women have the right one-to-one care, they are less likely to have this level of difficulty. In general, in our patriarchal society, there is a lack of investment in supporting women's health, and women's pain is routinely dismissed.

Because society doesn't get what breastfeeding is really like

I was on my knees with exhaustion and my mother kept telling me just to stop breastfeeding now because I'd done enough and it was time to stop with this silliness. If I stopped breastfeeding she assured me he would start sleeping through the night. In the end I gave in as after all she had four babies and she told me it worked for me and all my siblings. It didn't work and instead of feeding him back to sleep each time he woke I was pacing the room and trying to get him to take a dummy he

didn't want. I felt I'd lost my way to comfort him and felt so
guilty every time he cried knowing he could have been settled
if I could still feed him.

Society just doesn't 'get' babies. It doesn't seem to understand that they are helpless little mammals with frequent needs. It believes babies should be 'good' – sleep through the night, feed in a routine and be happy to be put down. And the messages that women get from society imply that they are failures if their baby breaks the rules.

There are so many myths out there. Formula will help your baby sleep (it won't). Put your baby in a feeding routine (it probably won't work and can reduce your milk supply). He's too clingy, you need to be stricter (he can barely lift his own head, you're his safe place). And so on. In so many women's stories they are convinced (by family, by books, by the formula industry) that if they just try to put their baby into a routine/give him formula/put him down then all their 'problems' will go away.[13]

All these seeming 'solutions' chip away at breastfeeding bit by bit, gradually reducing milk supply and resulting in a situation in which women feel they have to stop breastfeeding because they have no milk. Numerous research studies show that when you try to put a baby into a feeding routine and feed them less often or at a set time, women end up with less milk and are more likely to end up stopping breastfeeding. If you know how breastfeeding works, this makes a lot of sense. Milk is produced on a 'demand and supply' basis in that the baby 'demands' (asks nicely) for milk, and the more milk that is removed from the breast, the more milk gets made to replace it. Anything that reduces how much milk is removed from the breast can reduce how much milk the body makes, slowly reducing supply as the body thinks not much milk is needed.[14]

But how many messages are out there about putting your

baby in a routine? How many books suggest that babies can feed at set times? How many people actually realise that babies feeding frequently – e.g. every two hours or more – can be absolutely normal? Breastmilk is digested easily, and breastfed babies often prefer to feed little and often according to appetite. But when mothers do this and feed their baby responsively (e.g. whenever their baby wants to be fed) I can almost guarantee they'll find at least one person who tells them that they haven't got enough milk and something is wrong. This predictably leads to a formula top-up being offered, or a belief that babies can be taught to feed in a routine – which of course can then reduce milk supply, compounding the issue.[15]

So mothers end up with no milk and miserable, both because whatever they were promised would work didn't, and because they've ended up stopping breastfeeding before they are ready. And all through no fault of their own. Why are these messages allowed to be perpetuated? Where is the detailed antenatal education around how often babies feed and the damage that can be done if you try to interfere too much with that? Why are books promising that routines work still on the shelves? Why are so called 'experts' who repeat this message still sitting on television sofas?

Because society doesn't look after its new mothers

> *I so wanted to breastfeed him but it came to a point where I realised if I didn't get a break I was going to crack. What good was a mother who couldn't function to him even if he was getting breastmilk? Everyone kept telling me I needed to stop breastfeeding and put myself first now and eventually I believed them. But the awful part in all of this was that stopping didn't help at all and for a long time I just felt worse and angry at myself for having been so selfish.*

We are living in an age in which new mothers are the most isolated they have ever been. It wasn't meant to be this way. We weren't meant to have babies alone. We weren't meant to literally be left holding the baby, caring for them in isolation with no one really caring for us in return. The dispersal of western families means that many new parents have little experience or understanding of caring for a newborn, leaving many of us feeling a whole range of emotions once left to care for this brand new person alone. It's absolutely normal to feel shocked, overwhelmed, and even regretful. Of course this is all made a million times worse by feeling isolated.[16]

In women's responses to the research it was heartbreaking to see how many really were at breaking point. They often had very little day-to-day support. Sure, many had partners, but they were out all day and seemed to devolve any baby care to the mother even when they were home. Mothers were often used to being in good jobs, with a routine and interaction with others, and now they were in the house all day going from feed to feed feeling like their future would never be any different. Some were 'just' feeling isolated and exhausted, while others had been diagnosed with postnatal depression (and let's face it – when you're isolated and exhausted, depression has an open door to push against).

Critically, a central theme was that whenever women turned to others for help, breastfeeding was blamed. If they just stopped breastfeeding it would all be okay. They'd feel less overwhelmed. Their mental health challenges would magically disappear. Apparently all their difficulties were down to breastfeeding and once that was out of the way, they would be fine. Of course, often not much changed when they stopped. The reason so many women were overwhelmed in the first place was that they didn't have support circles around them. Their baby still needed feeding and settling to sleep and now they had lost the mothering tool of being able to breastfeed a fractious baby.

And on top of all this they then mourned the loss of their breastfeeding experience.

Because of others' beliefs and insecurities

We are social creatures and the attitudes, experiences and beliefs of those in our family and close to us affect how we feel and behave. And even though we might not realise it, the experiences of those around us affect how we feed our babies. This might not be obvious – it might be subtle behaviours and small actions that slowly damage breastfeeding for women, or persuade them that others should be involved in feeding the baby.[17]

When a woman is surrounded by those who have had positive experiences of breastfeeding, she is more likely to breastfeed for longer. If she was breastfed – and if her partner was breastfed – then she is more likely to be able to breastfeed. This isn't down to some biological quirk, but more the knowledge and attitudes of those around her. If they have experience of supporting breastfeeding they can help her with any challenges. They are likely to welcome her feeding and value it. They will know what helps and where to get help if needed.

Sadly, many women today have the opposite experience. This is compounded by generational experiences. Back in the 1950s we were sold the idea that formula milk was scientifically superior to breastfeeding and freed women from being tied to their babies. More and more mothers chose to bottle-feed, meaning that generational knowledge of breastfeeding was lost. There is a saying that 'breastfeeding is caught, not taught', meaning that if you grow up around breastfeeding, seeing how it works, and give birth in a community that knows how to help you, then you will be better prepared to breastfeed. Unfortunately, this lost generation informed the next generation, and so on… and now, even though our breastfeeding rates are much higher, many women have key women in their family who didn't breastfeed.[18]

Why does this matter? Those women may have a belief that bottle-feeding is better for the baby, or that it will help reduce the pressure. They may not know how to support a woman with breastfeeding difficulties, or they may give advice best suited to a bottle-fed baby. Some may deliberately try to sabotage breastfeeding – perhaps because they feel bottle-feeding is best, or because they couldn't breastfeed and don't want the mother to either. Some may be grieving their own difficulties breastfeeding, or the fact that they were persuaded not to, and consciously or subconsciously they find themselves harming their daughters' chances, passing on an inter-generational trauma. Those who did not breastfeed, or felt they had to do so discreetly, may feel uncomfortable with their daughter doing so in front of others or publicly.[19]

Another key figure is a mother's partner. Again, if they are supportive she is more likely to find it easier, and vice versa. Although much of the research into partner support has focused on the role of fathers, it is likely that some influences can be generalised to same-sex couples – albeit with some different challenges involved.[20]

My partner really didn't like me feeding her as he said he felt helpless and left out. He tried to pretend he wanted to give a bottle to help me but really he just wanted to feed her too. I let him persuade me that he could just do one feed at night but soon I found him giving more and when I asked him he'd say well it's my baby too. I think this was why I ended up not having enough milk for her and I really wish I had put a stop to it at the start as part of me really resents him now.

Unfortunately, many fathers report challenges in supporting breastfeeding. They are often excluded from antenatal breastfeeding education and feel unprepared when their partner has problems. They can want to fix things but feel helpless. Some can feel excluded and worry that they are not bonding with their baby, with some feeling embarrassed about her feeding in front of others. Some might see their partner struggling and feel bottle-feeding would be easier and more convenient.[21]

Although most fathers say they respect the mother's decision about how to feed their baby, some directly or indirectly sabotage her ability to do so. They might try to persuade her to let them give a bottle, either for their own involvement or because they think it will help her. They might make her feel uncomfortable feeding in front of others, or even put pressure on her about how she uses her body, claiming that it is 'theirs'. The growing involvement of fathers in caring for their babies is a good thing, but at the same time we are also seeing a growing number of fathers wanting to do everything for their baby, including feeding them.

Because the public can be idiots
It's 2019 as I write this and still we have the situation where women are being told that they can't breastfeed their babies in public places despite breastfeeding in any location being protected by law.[22] We still see women told to leave cafés. We still hear of women being openly criticised by someone in a restaurant. We still have tabloid readers commenting that they don't urinate in public.

Survey after survey shows us that women are made to feel uncomfortable, with some avoiding feeding in public at all. In the last UK Infant Feeding Survey, just 58% of mothers reported ever breastfeeding in public, with many feeling very self-conscious and worried that they were going to be approached and told to stop. Only 8% reported that they felt comfortable

85

breastfeeding whenever and wherever they liked.[1]

Of course, if you want to have any sort of life outside the house, feeding your baby in public is going to be part of that. So women who feel uncomfortable end up hiding in toilets, trying to feed in the car or cutting their trip short. It's understandable that they turn to formula milk when out and about or decide the whole thing is just too difficult and stop altogether.

Because maternity leave provision doesn't go far enough
Although many women in the UK benefit from paid maternity leave, not all women qualify and many return to work while breastfeeding a young baby, whether that is weeks or months after the birth. In other countries entitlement can be far less, with no state entitlement at all to maternity leave in the US. Not all maternity leave includes protection of breastfeeding once mothers are back in the workplace.

In the UK women do have some legal rights in the workplace when breastfeeding. They should have somewhere safe to rest, which should include a space to lie down, and a risk assessment should be carried out to make sure that the environment is safe to work in. However, making sure there is a private place to express milk, and a fridge to store it, is only 'recommended guidance', meaning many women find their employers will not support them in this way.[22]

Furthermore, women often report that their employers are at best shocked and at worst hostile when they make a request for support to continue breastfeeding. Some feel they are looked down upon or considered to not be fully engaged with their job.[23]

Because formula milk promotion is everywhere
Everyone thinks that formula milk advertising doesn't affect them, but it must be affecting somebody or the industry wouldn't bother pumping $9 billion every year into advertising. Although in the UK formula companies are not allowed to advertise their

products for babies under six months, in many countries such as the USA this is allowed and formula companies send samples and information to pregnant and new mothers whether they ask for it or not. And these free samples make a difference. A Cochrane review found that women who are given free samples of formula milk are less likely to continue breastfeeding.[24]

In the UK formula companies get around this by promoting formula for older babies, because they know that brand advertising means that sales of other products will increase too, and anyway, many people do not realise adverts for milks for older babies aren't promoting formula for younger babies.[25] In the UK Infant Feeding Survey, a third of mothers did not realise that there was a difference between infant formula and follow-on milk, with some even believing follow-on formula milk must be more nutritious.[1]

One reason why this promotion works is that formula companies don't just promote their products as straightforward milk for babies. They put a lot of money into adverts that suggest their specific brand will affect infant development, health, digestion and even sleep. They have careful adverts aimed at fathers, showing them cradling the baby while their partner sleeps blissfully. They sell the dream – the dream of a contented, quiet, sleeping baby.

The omnipresence of advertising also means that it targets *everyone*. It is everywhere. Fathers see it. Grandmothers see it. Friends see it. And even health professionals see it, because formula companies are allowed to sponsor events for health professionals as long as they are 'educational'.

All these reasons are why we owe it to women to make things better. They want to breastfeed, yet when they try to do so they face layer upon layer of obstacles in their way, all of which make women think it is actually their own fault that they cannot breastfeed.[13] And as described earlier, this is further tangled up in layers of social, cultural and racial inequalities, meaning that the women and babies who would benefit the most from breastfeeding often experience these barriers more harshly, coupled with also being least likely to get the professional support that they need.[26]

We need to do two things about this. First of all we need to carry on loudly pointing out all these issues, supporting women to see that they are not failing, but instead are being failed by the environment around them. Secondly, we need to crack on with changing the world, so that the next generation of women are not let down so badly.

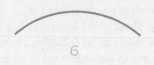

6

Healing from your own breastfeeding experience

We've covered what breastfeeding means to women, how they feel when they can't and why so many end up feeling so awful about the whole thing. So what can you do if you're struggling with your own emotions around breastfeeding, or supporting someone else?

The first step is to say that if you are feeling very strong emotions and are worried about your mental health, particularly if you strongly identify with the chapters discussing postnatal depression and trauma, please do seek professional support. This might be a GP, a counsellor or a private psychologist who specialises in trauma and grief. More on what you might expect from them a little later in this chapter.

Grief, however, is a spectrum. And if you are feeling any of the emotions discussed in this book (or indeed anything else), there are several things that might help if you are struggling to come to terms with your breastfeeding experience or how it ended. Each of these might be right for different people in different circumstances, so think about how you feel and whether (and who) you might feel comfortable speaking to about it. There will be no one right way for everyone.

1. Recognise how normal your feelings are

If you're grieving about your breastfeeding experience I can sadly bet that you have people telling you it just doesn't matter, or not even pausing to consider that it might. We know that most mean well. When people tell you that the main thing is that your baby is fed, they either don't realise how important breastfeeding is to you, or genuinely think it will help. Some may be comforted by these words, but for others it can make things worse.

With other losses, such as the death of a loved one, people recognise the importance of the loss and there are rituals and traditions as part of the grieving process. Yet with breastfeeding grief, you're just expected to get on with things. It's important that you recognise your emotions and give yourself time to grieve. Miriam Labbok, in her work on breastfeeding grief, spoke about the importance of treating this grief like any other grief and taking time and care of yourself to work through the different emotions.[1] Theories of grief acknowledge that everyone's response to a loss is different, with people feeling and responding differently. There is no one right way to feel or one right way to act.

Models that look at grief often talk about five stages, but in reality these describe five different things grieving people go through, rather than laying out a set order in which they happen. These include denial and feeling numb (trying to block out what happened), anger (at yourself or others), bargaining (could I have done something differently?), depression (sadness, regret, longing, despair) and finally, hopefully, some kind of acceptance. It is easy to recognise those different stages and reactions in women's stories.[2]

So take time to recognise how you feel, know that it is justified and normal and that over time, your feelings will start to change. They won't necessarily go away, but like any grief, they will change and adapt to your different stage in life. For some, this may be as you move out of the baby stage and there is less focus on breastfeeding, so if you are still in those early days, know that this is a possibility.

Likewise, if you're supporting someone through grief, recognise how important these feelings are to hear and acknowledge. Just being there, actively listening and supporting, can make all the difference. La Leche League has a useful leaflet here: www.laleche.org.uk/five-ways-help-breastfeeding-doesnt-go-expected

2. Be kind to yourself

It is so easy, as we can see from all the women's stories we've discussed, to blame ourselves when things go wrong. We think that if only had we tried a little harder or done something else then things might be different. Firstly, it's very easy to think like this with the benefit of hindsight, and secondly, we know that when a woman cannot breastfeed, her experience is rarely straightforward. If you're blaming yourself, ask – did I really get all the professional support I needed, including medical testing and diagnosis if things weren't working physically? Did my family really support me? Did my partner really do everything they could to help? Was I supported and valued as a mother trying to breastfeed her baby? What information and advice was I given from people who I trusted?

In the vast majority of cases women have been let down at least on one of these points. We do not live in a society that values, accepts and protects breastfeeding mothers. We set them up to fail – subtly and more directly – by placing numerous barriers in their way. Never ever feel that you have not done the 'best' for your baby. You have – it is just that what is best for your baby and family turned out to be different from what you'd hoped.

For other women their body simply didn't work, but they end up internalising the blame for this because there is often no medical reason given to explain what happened. When breastfeeding doesn't work for physiological reasons it is no more your fault than it is if your eyesight isn't perfect, but there are tests for that and we all accept not everyone has 20-20 vision.

In her book on birth trauma, Dr Emma Svanberg talks about an exercise she has developed called 'the perfect nurturer' to work with mothers who have traumatic memories of birth.[3] This exercise fits very well with working through feelings of breastfeeding grief. In this exercise she asks you to think about the kindest, warmest, most caring person that you either know or can imagine. This person is a real nurturer – they can see the bigger picture and respond gently and kindly to anything you say.

Then, whenever you find yourself feeling ashamed or guilty, ask yourself – what would they say? Would they go 'Oh yeah, actually Betty, you're sooo guilty here,' or would they kindly point out everything you had tried to do and how you were now caring for your baby? Because remember – breastfeeding is just one bit of caring for a baby. If you're blaming yourself and thinking you're a 'bad mother' then I bet you are not. You care for and love your baby in many, many different ways. That isn't to say that breastfeeding wasn't important to you, but always remember your baby is being loved and cared for in the very best way for you and your family.

Finally, know that you are not alone in this. Sadly, if you haven't been able to breastfeed as long as you wanted and you are grieving, you are one of a club that is growing every day. So many women are being let down. It's not just you. It's not just that you didn't try. It's a systemic issue that is bringing many women to their knees. Blame the system, not yourself.

3. Talk to someone

Talking about how you feel can be very cathartic. This might be as simple as opening up to a friend who you know will understand, or you might prefer to reach out to someone who is professionally trained in support, listening or counselling. It might be telling friends and family that this matters to you and why. It might be speaking out in a more public way, sharing your experiences and emotions. It might be blogging, privately or anonymously.

However, it is worth thinking about who you talk to. If breastfeeding was important to you, you might want to be cautious about sharing how you feel with anyone or any organisation that you think might give a 'the main thing is your baby is fed' message. Sometimes friends and family are best placed for these conversations and other times they're not (or you might prefer some additional support). There are a few places you can go for help.

Remember that breastfeeding support organisations are not just there for women who are breastfeeding. An important part of their work is to support women who have not been able to breastfeed for as long as they wanted. They can help you by talking through how you feel, and helping you work through what may have led you to this point – emphasising the point that breastfeeding is affected by so many things. It is not your fault that your breastfeeding experience was so challenging. I spoke to Justine Fieth, director of La Leche League GB, about the support they and other breastfeeding organisations provide. She explained:

> *In LLLGB, we often meet or talk with mothers who have gone to amazing lengths to try to make breastfeeding work. Some are still breastfeeding, some are combination-feeding and some are no longer breastfeeding. LLL Leaders can provide a*

listening ear for parents to talk about their feelings, concerns and experiences, enabling them to discuss their experience without judgement and supporting them in planning their future breastfeeding journeys.

La Leche League breastfeeding counsellors offer information and support to empower parents to make a decision that is right for them. We don't offer 'advice', as every mother/baby relationship is unique and what works for one may not be right for another. Often, having a chance to talk about a difficult breastfeeding experience with a breastfeeding counsellor can help to process and understand what happened and help parents find a sense of peace. And with that, many go on to have very different experiences with subsequent babies. You can contact an LLL Leader and your nearest group via **www. laleche.org.uk.**

Alternatively, you might want to consider talking privately to a lactation consultant about your experiences, particularly if you had a breastfeeding complication that led to you stopping. Again, they would be very well placed to help you explore what happened to you and how you are now feeling. They are not only there to make breastfeeding work, but take a holistic woman-centred approach to infant feeding as a whole. They can also support you with any queries you have about bottle-feeding and formula.

Another option might be to talk to a doula. You might think doulas are focussed on supporting women through birth, but postnatal support and talking to women is a key part of their role. I spoke to Maddie McMahon, doula trainer, breastfeeding counsellor and writer, about why a doula might be a great option for talking through your feelings. She explained:

Most postnatal doulas quickly find that they become adept at listening with attention and without judgement. It is a skill that is taught on our initial preparation course and honed with each client as they tell and re-tell their stories. Despite a widespread assumption that it is only the birth experience that can leave a mother with feelings of trauma and grief, I think most doulas would agree that it is often the narrative around infant feeding that ripples through motherhood most profoundly.

While doulas are not trained counsellors, and not all of us are lactation specialists, it is absolutely at the core of doula support to offer a form of therapeutic listening that can be cathartic and validating. But as well as just hearing a mother's emotions and empathising, a doula's superpower is signposting. With their finger on the birth and breastfeeding pulse, it is likely your doula will be able to point you towards local and national services and people that can support parents as they come to a place of peace.

You don't have to have had a birth doula or even an existing postnatal doula to access the unconditional, non-judgemental support of a doula. If you feel the need to unburden yourself, reach out to any doula in your area by putting your postcode into **www.doula.org.uk.**

There are also a number of specialist midwives, health visitors and other birth and parenting experts who are now providing specific listening and counselling options for those experiencing breastfeeding grief. Have a look online (paying careful attention to qualifications and testimonials before paying any money) at the range of help and support now out there.

Some specialists have been seeing positive outcomes using something called the 'three-step rewind technique'. I must stress at this point that there isn't much published evidence into its impact, but those who have received support through such therapy do seem to find it has a positive impact on their feelings and memories, particularly around trauma and grief related to birth and feeding. I spoke to Ros McFadden, a lactation consultant who offers these services through the Breastfeeding Hub MK **www.breastfeedinghub.org/courses-workshops.**

THE THREE STEP REWIND TECHNIQUE

What support do you offer women who are experiencing grief and trauma?

As a registered midwife and an International Board Certified Lactation Consultant (IBCLC), I offer private one-to-one consultations and run a voluntary community drop-in breastfeeding café. An integral part of my initial history-taking in either of these settings will be to gain an insight into experiences leading up to the present. The partner is often present and the way they tell their story often highlights whether certain events have triggered traumatic feelings and responses.

As a health professional I may perceive a birth experience or event as traumatic, but it may not be deemed so by the parent and vice versa. Trauma is how a person processes an experience. The heightened emotions present during a trauma, instead of being filed as a past event in the hippocampus, are recorded directly in the amygdala (our alarm system mobilising our fight, flight or freeze response), embedding the emotional response in the memory of the event or period of time.

The programme I offer to support those who have experienced trauma is based on techniques that enable them to process their thoughts and re-programme the way in which they react to the event in the future.

What does that involve?

The technique I have been trained to teach clients is the Three -Step Rewind Process, which uses deep relaxation, visualisation techniques and outcome-focused questions to establish how they wish to feel in the future. The client does not have to reveal their story if they find it too distressing to do so, and this is client led, but some may find sharing cathartic. The programme is generally run over three sessions, working through each step in sequence.

In the initial step the client is asked to score how they feel using the Subjective Unit of Distress (SUD) scale where 0 is no feeling and 10 is very highly distressed. The aim is to establish a safe place for the client to share their story or think about what happened without sharing, while the practitioner uses empathetic listening skills. I would note the descriptive words used when recalling the event and their distressing symptoms, and how they would like to feel in the future when talking of or thinking about the event, using the outcome-focused questions. The session concludes with a deep relaxation, which I often record for them to use at home, and they rescore using the SUD scale.

Step two involves an initial SUD score, giving an idea of any improvement, the deep relaxation process is repeated and this time leads into the rewind process. The rewind process is a form of visualisation of the event or period of time played through in the client's mind, rewound, played forward again, rewound and finally played forward while visualising the future. Again the session ends with a SUD rescore.

In step three the initial score determines whether the full rewind process needs repeating if there hasn't been enough of an improvement. The process concludes with repeating the deep relaxation, reframe and building the future visualisations.

How does it work?
The deep relaxation involves the client visualising their place of relaxation. Once in this deep relaxed state they are receptive to beginning the process, which starts with the Double Disassociated Rewind – playing their story while watching

themselves watching the film play out. When the film reaches the end, they are asked to rewind the film really fast. Next is the Disassociated Rewind – watching the film play out in front them, then rewinding fast when it completes. The final stages are: Associated Rewind, where the client enters the film and experiences the film first hand, including the fast rewind; Reframe involving removing a DVD of their film and disposing of it, reconnected with their place of relaxation; and the Building the Future stage, where a film of the client in the future plays out and they experience the feelings they identified in their outcome-focussed question replies, creating a 'blueprint' for their future.

The theory behind the process is that the client can detach the associated emotions of the trauma from the memory. They are still able to remember the event, but it has now been stored in their long-term memory where they are able to rationally process it.

How do women feel afterwards?

I find clients have differing levels of SUD score during and after the process. Most see an improvement at the end of sessions one and two, but some may need to repeat the full process on the third visit. All have found that the process helped them be in control of the memory.

Ideally a parent will work through this process before they attend any 'Birth Afterthoughts' meetings where they are given the opportunity to go over their notes and the birth. By learning the process first, they will be less likely to trigger severe distressing emotions. I am finding that parents seek this support as they are planning their next baby, or the mother is pregnant again. This could be because the distressing emotions have been triggered by the thought of a repetition. I would recommend they seek support in learning this technique sooner rather than later. The power of this technique has driven me to ask a fellow practitioner to help me work through the technique for my own trauma.

4. Take care of yourself

One of the core approaches to helping people who are experiencing grief, trauma or anxiety and depression (or all of them at once) is not only to explore why it has happened and how they feel, but also to help them cope with any symptoms they are experiencing. So when anger, anxiety or depressive symptoms crop up, the person has a number of cognitive coping strategies in place to help them. Effectively it is looking at symptom management alongside the core root of those symptoms.[4,5] Although everyone is different and will benefit in different ways, some of the ideas you might like try include:

- Being active and getting outside. Nature is restorative and if you are experiencing anxiety and feeling on edge then exercise can help burn off adrenaline and release feel-good endorphins. Try and focus on your body as you move – feel the movement, your heart rate and notice your surroundings.
- Try not to shut yourself off from everyone. Choose your friends and contacts carefully, but don't completely isolate yourself. As above, talk about how you feel to someone who will listen. For some volunteering can help – perhaps supporting one of the breastfeeding or trauma organisations. Or try something completely different and new.
- Try to calm your system. Relaxation exercises such as breathing and noticing things around you can help calm you down. Comfort yourself. Do you have a favourite smell, taste, place, piece of music or clothing that helps relax you? Might yoga or meditation help

you? For some people, keeping a diary and writing down their thoughts helps. For others, relaxing tasks that keep your mind distracted are useful – jigsaws, painting, colouring, knitting and so on.

- Challenge your negative thoughts. Are they really true? Imagine a friend was telling you the same things. What would you say to them?
- Try to look after your health. You know the drill. Plenty of sleep, a balanced diet, watch the alcohol.

An excellent practical guide to taking steps to overcome any negative emotions you are feeling about your infant feeding experience is the work of Hilary Jacobsen. Hilary is a holistic breastfeeding consultant and hypnotherapist and has written a book called *Healing Breastfeeding Grief*, which explores lots of different techniques that can help you work through the emotions you may be feeling. The book aims to help mothers understand their emotions and where they came from and find ways of moving forward.

Hilary has a particular focus on calming the anxiety that can be a big part of breastfeeding grief. She has a number of exercises that can be done almost anywhere to help you slow down racing thoughts and calm a jittery mind and body. You can find out more about Hilary's work on her webpage www. healingbreastfeedinggrief.com or her Facebook page www. facebook.com/breastfeedingmomgrief.

5. *Consider giving feedback*
If you are in the depths of grief, this may not be an option that is right for you at the moment. But as you move forward, you might want to think about how your experiences could be used to better support women in the future. Your hospital should have its own Patient Advice and Liaison Service (PALS) or

Maternity Voices Partnership (MVP), which you can use to feedback and/or complain about care received.

You might even want to consider training with one of the breastfeeding organisations yourself to support more women in the future. You might be surprised to know that many of today's peer supporters, breastfeeding counsellors and lactation specialists are not in their roles purely because they had an easy, fabulous time breastfeeding – but in fact because they experienced the exact opposite. Many had difficult experiences and stopped breastfeeding before they were ready, or needed to use formula when they didn't want to. They get it. They've been there. They understand.

Seeking professional support

If you are experiencing very strong emotions, particularly if they are getting in the way of your day-to-day life, or perhaps affecting how much you are able to sleep or relax, please do think about seeking some specialised support with your feelings. Anxiety, depression and anger are very common symptoms in the months after having a baby and can be exacerbated by feelings of trauma related to your pregnancy, birth or feeding experiences. As you may well know, these things can all get intertwined and tied up together, and it can be difficult trying to pinpoint what exactly is causing you to feel distressed – or indeed even how you are feeling. But there are people out there who can help, whether it is a more generalised approach to trauma or specific to your experiences.

If you are unsure about how strong your feelings are, or are worrying that they are not 'serious enough' to take up the time of a professional, it might be worth reflecting on some of the questions a professional might use to assess whether someone is experiencing clinical anxiety or depression. The Hospital Anxiety and Depression scale[6] is one such tool and asks individuals to reflect on statements such as:

- I feel tense or wound up
- I feel as if I am slowed down
- I get a sort of frightened feeling like butterflies in the stomach
- I get a sort of frightened feeling as if something awful is about to happen
- I have lost interest in my appearance
- I feel restless as if I have to be on the move
- Worrying thoughts go through my mind
- I get sudden feelings of panic

If you think you are experiencing symptoms such as these, or indeed the feelings listed in the earlier trauma section of the book, and are also struggling to feel relaxed and happy about things that usually make you happy, please do contact your GP or a private counsellor.

Unfortunately, there is not a lot of research into specifically supporting women to process trauma and grief related to their breastfeeding experience. However, many of the processes used for supporting women with more generalised trauma, anxiety or depression are likely to be helpful, especially with a counsellor or psychologist who really understands the importance of breastfeeding to you. Any good counsellor will of course not judge whether someone's grief or trauma is 'worthy', but it is important to know that they understand. Finding someone who specialises in mental health related to birth and motherhood is likely to be a very good first step.

In terms of which specific therapies might help, again there is very little research into what might help with breastfeeding grief or trauma. It is important to know that for more significant grief and trauma, there is little evidence that simple debriefing (talking about your experience) helps,[7] without the use of therapy to help you work through it. Talking may help if you are 'just' dealing with some difficult feelings, but if you are experiencing clinical trauma symptoms such as not being able to sleep, or the scale of your feelings is impacting on your day-to-day life, it is important to find an evidence-based approach to helping the trauma heal.

Two approaches[8] that have been shown to help individuals deal with trauma are Cognitive Behavioural Therapy (CBT), which involves helping an individual reattribute meaning to what happened to them, and Eye Movement Desensitization and Reprocessing (EMDR), a psychotherapy technique which helps the individual move memories from being stuck in the present, to being part of their past. You might like to look up individuals who specialise in these therapies, or ask your GP what types of counselling might be available. This is not to say that other forms of counselling do not work, just that there is an evidence base for these two approaches working for trauma experiences.

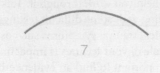

7

What can we do to make things better?

Finally, what can we actually do to improve things for future generations? Of course, recognising how women feel when they are not able to breastfeed and supporting them is part of the solution, but there's also what we can do to try and ensure that fewer women feel this way in the first place.

Importantly, this must not jeopardise breastfeeding support, especially for those living in more marginalised groups, for whom breastfeeding may be one of the most accessible ways they have of protecting their baby's health. We must not shy away from talking about the importance of breastfeeding, but perhaps we can do it differently. We need to think bigger than the idea of 'breastfeeding versus formula feeding'. We need to make sure:

1. That every woman who wants to breastfeed, and can physiologically breastfeed, is given the very best chance of doing so.
2. That women who want to breastfeed but cannot

breastfeed have support, information and choices.

3. That no woman is made to feel guilty or a failure because of her infant feeding experiences – especially when she has been let down by others.

4. That we listen to women and help them heal.

This will be a big job.

No single action is going to change things for new mothers overnight. But we have lots of ideas. As part of my research I asked women what they would like to see change. Some said that they didn't have any ideas, but they hoped that something could be done to change things for others. Others noted that although they felt pain when breastfeeding was discussed, they didn't want this to be a reason for fewer conversations about breastfeeding or others being supported. They felt that although it hurt them, they could see why it was needed. Others had clear ideas about what we need to do to make things better, based on supporting women better when they cannot breastfeed, and also making sure fewer women in the future feel this way.

From their responses, two things stood out to me. Firstly, that many women who were hurting deeply were still suggesting solutions for better supporting breastfeeding in the future. And secondly, that although women were mourning their breastfeeding relationships, a lot of what they suggested could help them was based on their treatment when they couldn't breastfeed. Women often described how a lot of the hurt they experienced came not just from being unable to breastfeed, but also from how they felt they were viewed, and treated, once they had make the decision to stop.

While we can't necessarily overcome huge societal barriers to ensuring breastfeeding women are supported overnight, making smaller changes to how women are treated when they're struggling is surely easier.

What did women suggest?

1. Better support for breastfeeding

Women were hurting, angry and grieving, yet the very first thing many said was that they wished there was better support for breastfeeding in the first place. They had been deeply let down by a lack of support, but hoped that women in the future would not experience these issues. Importantly, this idea of 'more support' was broad and complex. It didn't just mean a little extra practical support, but overhauling the whole system.

Women particularly wanted to see:

a) More skilled support

Women wanted more availability of skilled support so that problems they experienced could be identified sooner, rather than, as was often the case, being told there was no issue. Specifics included issues like recognition of weight loss, tongue tie and allergies.

> *Not enough is done to combat issues such as tongue tie. It took 13 weeks for doctors to resolve my son's posterior tie, so when women are struggling they get told to supplement with formula which leads to feelings of failure.*

Others wanted much broader support, raising the idea of ample, regular breastfeeding support clinics staffed by a range of professionals – just as you might attend for other health complications.

> *If I had all the money in the world, I would create breastfeeding clinics where mothers could sit for as long as needed to get into the swing of things.*

The key was the availability. Women didn't want to look up when their next local breastfeeding support group was and see it was five days away. They wanted to be able to go to one that day. And the next day. And for it to be open all day. Perhaps in some areas this sort of support is available. But in many places, funding for breastfeeding support has been slashed, leaving women with just one or two groups a week, or in some cases barely any at all.

b) Better training for professionals

Another thing that stood out from women's responses was a call for improved training for professionals, and not just those whose primary job it was to support breastfeeding day-to-day (such as midwives or health visitors), but also those whose advice and behaviour could have an impact on breastfeeding success.

> *Everyone who gives advice on breastfeeding or looking after a baby should know how to best support breastfeeding, especially if their information can affect whether a mother continues or not. This needs to include GPs who often give bad advice on different medications, but I think anyone who can cause difficulties should have basic knowledge at least, such as childcare workers.*

Sadly, we know that many medics have very little training on breastfeeding as part of their education, including paediatricians and GPs, although the most passionate and interested will find additional training and support. This means that women can end up receiving inaccurate or misleading advice. A recent evaluation we conducted for the Breastfeeding Network of their specialist pharmacist-led Drugs in Breastmilk information service showed just how often women were contacting the service after being told they could not breastfeed, for the simplest of medications such as antihistamines, anaesthetics and antibiotics. All of these are medications that the majority of women should be able to take while breastfeeding, or a suitable alternative found.[1]

Another common suggestion was that all midwives and health visitors should have advanced training as lactation consultants so that they are equipped to deal with complications as they arise. This may of course not be feasible, and an understanding of breastfeeding sufficient to spot a problem and refer to specialist services may be more useful. You do not need an entire system that has the top level of expertise. But consistency and skill are important.

c) Better diagnosis of complications

A strikingly frequent issue was the concept that when things did go wrong, not only, as above, were these issues often missed or dismissed, but even if a professional was supportive and taking the time to understand, there was simply no answer available. Women were often told that breastfeeding wasn't working, but were rarely given a 'diagnosis' or explanation for why, with many reporting that the usual approach appeared to be to tell them to just give formula as if that would solve all their problems.

> *For me, it wasn't so much not being able to breastfeed but that there was no reason given. It seemed to be that I should just accept I couldn't and move on and that felt ludicrous. I'd never visited a GP before and just been told there was no answer and to use an alternative. When I'd attended for far more minor issues I had been sent for a battery of tests, and now when this one thing that they had spent so much time telling me was vitally important wasn't working, there was nothing about it at all.*

Even if women were happy to give formula, and noted that their baby seemed fine on it, they were still angry that there had been no explanation. In her book *Unlatched*, Jennifer Grayson talks about her interview with Peter Hartmann, and the fact that in all these years of conducting research into the health outcomes of breastfeeding, so little investigation had been done into understanding *why* breastfeeding wasn't working.[2]

To return to a point I made earlier, can you imagine this happening to a man? He gets the courage up to go to the GP to talk about his erectile dysfunction (after having tried the myriad of readily available treatments available online and at pharmacist counters). He tells the GP his symptoms and how he's feeling and the GP responds *'Oh well, never mind, some men just can't. There are alternatives out there you could use. Next patient please!'* It simply wouldn't happen – and nor should it – but all around the world women are effectively told the same thing because there is a lack of funding and scientific investment in understanding the breast as a reproductive organ.

A lack of diagnosis also has further consequences. Many mothers explained how, in the absence of 'proof' or a diagnosis they could show people, they blamed themselves for not trying hard enough. Others felt that they were being judged by others who thought they could have continued, as there was no medical evidence for stopping.

The GP said in a matter-of-fact way that I wouldn't be making enough milk for him so to just move on to formula now as there was no point in doing both. I was kind of relieved in a way but also really anxious that no one would believe me. I don't know if I wanted a reason to be given for my own peace of mind or to tell others because I worried they wouldn't believe me and would think I just stopped for my own benefit.

Conversely, surprise surprise, those who had managed to get a physiological explanation for their difficulties felt relieved and that it was not their fault.

Of course, for more support to be possible we need investment. Investment in training and increased staffing so that people have enough time to spend with women, and specialists are available when needed. Investment at every level, from maternity support workers through to IBCLCs for more complex cases. Support this in the community with an array of feeding groups, from specific breastfeeding ones through to ones for all different types of feeding scenarios.

Changes to medical training should include an understanding of the role of infant feeding in determining health and disease over a life course, with an understanding of normal baby behaviour and the practicalities of supporting mothers to breastfeed as part of a multidisciplinary approach. The World Breastfeeding Trends Initiative (WBTI) indicator five, 'Health and nutrition care systems', sets out a full list of what a skilled breastfeeding support workforce would look like.[3]

2. Be honest about what breastfeeding is really like
Breastfeeding might be natural and normal and all those words, but that doesn't make it easy. Just as it often takes time to develop any other physical skill (such as crawling or walking), it can take time to get the hang of breastfeeding. It might look as straightforward as just latching that baby on the breast, but a whole load of factors are often against us, from a stressful birth to being in an uncomfortable position through to barely having seen anyone else breastfeed so we are less instinctively aware of how to hold and position our baby.

Breastfeeding is more than just latching the baby on. It's about understanding normal baby behaviour: how much they feed (lots), how much they sleep (little) and how much they like being put down (basically never) and then how building milk supply and responsive frequent feeding build into all of that to make breastfeeding work. But how often are we taught all of this in antenatal classes? And how often do the friends and family around us know this information and support us throughout it?

Be more honest about the realities of breastfeeding. For most women it is not immediately straightforward and this coming as a shock makes it harder to deal with and I believe leads more women to stop as they do not expect problems or know where to turn and can feel very alone.

For many first-time mothers, the reality is the opposite. Strangers go on about good babies. Adverts promise your baby will sleep through the night. Books tell you that you can get your baby in a routine and get your life back. And where does that leave you when your baby refuses to cooperate? Wondering where it all went wrong, when nothing is really 'wrong' at all apart from the story you were told and a lack of support.

A big part of this is thinking about problem-solving and spotting complications before they get too far. Many women talked about attending antenatal classes but not being taught about the complications to look out for. This meant they often didn't seek help in the early stages, or didn't realise something was fixable.

Just make sure mothers-to-be know exactly any single problem that can happen when trying to breastfeed and how to react quickly. It's easier to do this when pregnant than with a hungry baby crying next to a zombie mum in desperation. Did I know what thrush, mastitis, tongue tie was before having a baby? Not a clue! Did I attend a breastfeeding workshop? Yes! So why hiding all that information – it's outrageous.

We must make sure that more women have access to information and education that equips them to be able to breastfeed. Some people have told me that you can't tell women about complications or you will put them off breastfeeding. Hmmm. Well, for a start, they're just about to give birth and that's not usually a walk in the park. But second, what on earth are you saying about women here? That they won't do anything that might be a bit uncomfortable or challenging? As if the rest of motherhood is just really, really straightforward and full of fluffy marshmallows and unicorns or something?

We prepare ourselves for difficult situations all the time. When you take a driving test you learn how to spot hazards, change a tyre, do an emergency stop. Are we going to stop teaching people those in case it puts them off driving? Or might it just be better that they are informed and able in difficult situations?

> *Stop portraying breastfeeding as a utopia, then personal expectations may be lower. No one talks about what can go wrong or how long a feed can take.*

Most of all, it is easy to see why women are so angry at health services that let them down. To have to stop breastfeeding because you have some kind of health complication is difficult enough. But to be told you have to stop breastfeeding because of something that you then find out is fixable and you simply weren't given the right advice? That is soul-destroying and essentially medical negligence, surely. Can you imagine the uproar if people were not being told important information about their health for any other bodily function? There would rightly be an outcry, but again it's as if breastfeeding is seen by some as an 'optional extra' that you can just take or leave if it gets a bit tricky.

Finally, we must think about the inevitable consequences of repeatedly telling women that breastfeeding is straightforward and magical. If someone keeps telling you it's all great, really easy... and then you find it really tricky... what thoughts and doubts start to creep into your mind? That it must be your fault? That you didn't try hard enough? That you're not as tough as everyone else?

No, no and no!!

There are a whole range of breastfeeding experiences out there, from women who found it pretty easy to those who really struggled – all because their own personal breastfeeding experiences and contexts were different. Just like everything else in life.

3. Think about the words used in breastfeeding promotion strategies

Another key point is to think about the way we promote breastfeeding, in a world where so many women have been let down. Many women spoke about how the wording used in breastfeeding promotion messaging 'triggered' their negative emotions, making them react in a way they didn't necessarily want to. There were lots of different ideas women had for ways messages could be changed – not to alter the deeper content, but to change the words used, so they were less hurtful.

> There are ways of talking about breastfeeding that don't automatically demonise women who can't or don't. Please think more about the words used and how they might feel to someone who really wanted to breastfeed but could not.

Get rid of breast is best

Ugh, are we still using this one? This awful phrase is still seen across platforms, from policies to social media posts, even including the World Health Organization. I could write an entire book on this, but there are several reasons why I want to see the back of this phrase once and for all.

Best? As against what? Breastfeeding shouldn't have value judgements placed against it. It is what it is – a biologically normal way to feed milk to an infant.

Best? As in doing your best? No thank you. As one of the women pointed out in her quote above, whenever she heard it, it made her feel as though she was not doing her 'best', even when she very much wanted to breastfeed and had tried hard to do so but met too many barriers. Moving to formula, in her circumstances, was doing what was 'best' for her baby.

Best? As in best mother? Let's not even go there.

Most of all, although many women noted that they felt breastfeeding was technically 'best' for their infants, telling them something was best didn't in any way enable them to do it. Of course it didn't. If telling people something was best for them suddenly inspired and enabled them to immediately be able to do it, then we'd have no public health issues at all.

Why does the government think telling women something is best is in any way helpful? I know it's best but it misses the point that I AM trying my best.

Telling women breastfeeding is best and to get on with it also loads all the responsibility on to them, suggesting that if they wanted what was best for their baby they would do it. But this ignores all the societal barriers in their way… which damage their ability to breastfeed and then cleverly also make them blame themselves. Touché.

Stop suggesting it's all a choice

Choice. A small word with a lot of meaning. It makes is sound like such an easy selection doesn't it, of this array of positive possibilities. It makes it sound like something you wanted. Something you were responsible for choosing willingly over and above any other option.

Choice? It was never my choice! I would never choose this or to feel this way.

Some women talked about how the word 'decision' felt more suitable. It was a decision – a very difficult decision. This word felt like a more sober, considered word than the suggestions of frivolity and utopias brought about by the word 'choice'.

Stop saying that women 'give up' breastfeeding
Women do not give up breastfeeding. I repeat, they do not give up. They may decide to stop. They may get to the end of their tether. They may be forced into it. But at no point does a woman who wants to breastfeed go *'Oh you know, I can't be bothered with this, I'm chucking it all in'*.

> *Don't dare ever suggest I gave up breastfeeding. How can people say that? Like we just rolled over and abandoned it all? I stopped breastfeeding after four weeks of triple pumping. Feed the baby, top the baby up, express more milk for the baby and repeat over and over. I tried and tried but I just couldn't make enough for him. If four weeks of doing that and barely sleeping is giving up, well I don't know what to say.*

Giving up implies women have been defeated – that they weren't strong enough or dedicated enough to continue, again without recognising the sheer effort they had often expended to try and overcome barriers placed in their way.

Don't talk about 'failure to breastfeed'
That little F-word can be found throughout the birth and baby literature – castigating women when they are at their most vulnerable. Failure to progress. Failure to breastfeed. Imagine the same for men – erection failure anyone? Or are we gentler than that, more sensitive, knowing that these things are emotive and linked to identity?

> *I want to throttle anyone who uses the word failed when talking about a mother.*

Failure is the ultimate judgement word. You tried… but you

failed. Nope, I'm not having it. No woman fails when it comes to birth or feeding their baby. They most likely have *been failed.* Telling women that they 'failed' also places all responsibility on the mother. It's not us who failed you, by not funding the support you needed/making you go back to work too soon/making you feel really awkward about feeding your baby outside the house/ not identifying your problem soon enough… it's you… YOU! Society doesn't recognise that it was actually the system that failed, or we would have to do something about it…

Is it any wonder women feel so down when they can't breastfeed? Every phrase used to describe it stinks of judgement and personal responsibility. It's a form of gaslighting really. Telling a woman that she has failed to breastfeed when in fact the environment she was trying to breastfeed in made it impossible.

4. Look at the content of breastfeeding promotion materials
Women also made a number of suggestions about how the content of breastfeeding promotion might change. Although mothers recognised that messages highlighting the protective benefit of breastfeeding were important, they also felt that messages aimed only at highlighting the protection for the infant induced feelings of extreme responsibility and guilt for the mother, whereas other messages might be less problematic. For example, why do campaigns rarely focus on protection for the mother?

You rarely see posters saying how breastfeeding can help protect against things like breast cancer. Why not? I felt like breastfeeding only mattered for my baby, so formula was pushed on me as the solution as my baby would then be fed and I could then get a break as if this had no impact on me whatsoever. What about me and my reduced risk of breast cancer, why didn't this matter? Meanwhile I have friends who have been told they are just continuing to breastfeed for themselves, as if there was something wrong with that, it's crazy how little we seem to realise that breastfeeding helps women too.

Another issue with current messaging was the common use of deterministic language, which seemed to suggest that all formula-fed babies would automatically get ill. This is a big issue in public health at the moment: the importance of talking about risks in a sensible way. Public health messaging is often over-simplified to the point of being inaccurate. Barely anything in life when it comes to our health is directly determined by one simple thing. Plenty of people live to an old age while smoking and chucking back the whisky. Meanwhile, plenty of people who are much healthier die much sooner. It's all about numbers on a population level – numbers that were never meant to be applied to individuals, but are used by public health experts to spot patterns and identify where changes might be possible. Mothers wanted to know the *absolute risk* – what percentage of babies might get sick – rather than the *relative risk*, which sounds much scarier – 'five times the risk'.

Talk about the real risks rather than saying five times more likely. Five times what? That might just mean you have just a 5% risk, or in other words a 95% chance your baby still won't get it.

Another idea was that there often wasn't any need to refer to formula at all when you talked about the benefits of breastfeeding. A number of women felt that they started to get irritated with messages around breastfeeding that viewed formula negatively, or even demonised formula.

Don't shame women. In our local labour ward they have a poster displayed saying how breastfeeding reduces the risk of obesity. There are two images… one of a baby at the breast, one of a baby covered in Mars bar wrappers – that is a disgrace!

117

I really hope that promotion posters like these are few and far between. Surely anyone with a bit of common sense can see the issue with the imagery and suggestions on that poster? It can understandably lead to women feeling that they are doing harm to their baby if they need to formula feed, when of course, if their baby cannot be breastfed then it is important that they are formula fed rather than having cows' milk or other foods. You can promote all sorts of things without having to demonise the alternative. You can encourage people to get out and go for a walk, without demonising those sat on the sofa for the evening – recognising that there may be many, many reasons why they are sat there.

Finally, some women asked whether we actually needed to direct breastfeeding promotion messages at women at all. They described how they wanted to breastfeed, but the problems they faced were with everyone else: partners, family, the public, even employers. They have an excellent point. Breastfeeding is a public health level societal responsibility – not just something women do. Yet we keep directing messages at women, as if no one wants to breastfeed.

I know why breastfeeding is so important, you don't have to tell me. If you could have perhaps told my partner to support me better, or got my boss to give me a break, then perhaps I would still be breastfeeding now.

The idea that perhaps health promotion shouldn't really focus on women at all, instead concentrating on creating the environment around them which helps them to breastfeed, is now gaining traction. We must stop focusing solely on public health campaigns aimed at individual women and instead focus on those whose attitudes affect her – family, friends, employers and the general public. We know that the attitudes of those close to the mother and their willingness and ability to support her to breastfeed have a significant impact on her ability to continue. So why are we not including those people more widely in our breastfeeding promotion and support messages?

On a societal level, education is needed on infant feeding right through from the early years. College and university students hold some of the most negative views about breastfeeding. Surrounded by images of sexualised breasts and with little experience of infant care, breastfeeding is alien to them. Yet if they have grown up seeing breastfeeding, they are more likely to have positive attitudes.[4] Younger children see many images of bottles and babies in their books and home corners at school, but where are the images of babies breastfeeding? As they get older, where is breastfeeding on the curriculum? It is a natural step to include it in many subjects – biology, economics, nutrition, personal and social education and so on. If it were there, there would be far less need to promote it at a later stage.

Our public health messaging also needs to be more specific about how individuals can help support breastfeeding and why it is important, rather than promulgating vague alliterative slogans. As the *Lancet* series on breastfeeding in 2016 stated:

> *The success or failure of breastfeeding should not be seen solely as the responsibility of the woman. Her ability to breastfeed is very much shaped by the support and the environment in which she lives. There is a broader responsibility of governments and society to support women through policies and programmes in the community.*

5. Recognise the emotions that not being able to breastfeed can bring
This was a huge one. And it is unsurprising really. Many women described how they felt confused by the way they were treated when they needed to stop breastfeeding. All the way through their pregnancy they had been told that breastfeeding was really

important and that they should give it a go, and then when they couldn't... it suddenly didn't matter at all.

No one said anything at all. At one point I felt like screaming, is no one going to ask me if I'm ok here? Is no one going to recognise that this is something I really wanted to do and everyone told me was vital and now I can't?

Sometimes there was just a complete silence, as if no one had even contemplated that women would have any kind of emotional reaction to stopping breastfeeding. They were formula feeding now and that was that. A bit like deciding which type of apple to buy in the supermarket. You liked this type, but it was out of stock so you got a different type instead. Actually, no, forget that – some people might be more understanding if your favourite pink ladies were out of stock than if you'd stopped breastfeeding.

This lovely midwife said to me 'It really hurts, doesn't it?' and it made such a difference. I felt like someone had validated my feelings and recognised it was important to me. I needed to hear that and she helped me to heal.

Validation is important when it comes to emotions. Women wanted someone to see their pain and difficulty and acknowledge it, rather than pretending it didn't matter or exist. Just a few kind words made all the difference.

I am a strong believer that breastmilk is best but breastfeeding isn't always. Feeding is important but so is love and a mother who has it together. Recognise that sometimes a mum has to make a difficult decision when it comes to feeding that might seem wrong but actually is the right one for her family.

Others wanted reassurance that they were doing the right

thing for their baby by stopping breastfeeding, or that they were still doing well in caring for their baby in other ways, despite what they saw as a failure. If we fail to recognise the enormity of the emotion that not being able to breastfeed can bring, women do not receive the reassurance they so desperately need. We all benefit from being told we're doing a good job caring for our babies, don't we? And when we are feeling really low it can make all the difference if people are kind.

I think every mum who stops breastfeeding should be offered a debrief of some kind with someone who understands and knows how they are feeling.

A core part of this is to more formally and openly support women who have not been able to meet their infant feeding goals. We must be there for those who couldn't breastfeed or couldn't breastfeed for as long or as exclusively as they wanted to. We must challenge the notion that for many women, feeding their baby is not just about nutrition, it is so much more.

A service to support these women would recognise that every woman is unique and has different circumstances. And any support would be tailored to her unique perspective. We know even on a really simple level that the words that work to help some women heal will cause further damage in others.

1. What were her goals? What did she hope for?
2. How is she feeling – what specific emotions?
3. What does she wish was different?

In particular, if a health professional tells a woman she must use formula, there must be space and opportunity for this to be discussed, rather than a simple 'just give a bottle' as if it will not matter. Of course, some women will be fine – maybe they weren't particularly attached to breastfeeding, or are happy with their decision. Great. But many would value more consideration

121

– and that is absolutely fine too. Space must be created to debrief women who are grieving a loss or substantial difference in how they hoped their breastfeeding journey would look.

Is fed best?

This moves us directly onto the recent tendency to tell mums who haven't been able to breastfeed that it doesn't matter and 'fed is best'. I did not mention this phrase at all in the research questions, but the wording emerged from the data many times.

> *I find comfort in thinking that at least fed is best. My baby is ok and I am trying.*

Some mothers said they found the phrase comforting, feeling that it emphasised that the main thing was that their baby was fed, and that they were still caring for their baby despite not meeting their own expectations.

> *I despise this new tendency to tell mums that fed is best. Whenever someone says it I just feel like I'm wrong for feeling so strongly and they don't care how I feel.*

However, more mothers felt that the phrase, although often said with good intentions, actually made them feel worse. All they could hear was that no one cared about how they felt, and that the main thing was that their baby was fed… their emotions didn't matter and to feel anything negative was wrong, as this suggested they cared more about themselves than the baby.

> *I actually feel better when someone tells me they understand how I feel and if I had followed my instincts and not topped up she would have probably been fine. I feel really angry and have to bite my tongue when people tell me 'fed is best', as of course it's better than starving my baby, but nowhere near as good as breast.*

No one who feels breastfeeding is important to them is saying that they would rather their baby not be fed. Feeding the baby of course is the absolute bottom line! But do we not deserve more than the bottom line? For many, 'fed is best' feels like the equivalent of telling a new mother who has just given birth that all that matters is she has a healthy baby. Of course everyone wants a healthy baby. But these things aren't an either/or situation! It's not as though you get to pick one – your baby's health, or your happiness. You are allowed to be relieved and grateful that your baby is healthy and fed, but still be deeply grieving the loss of your breastfeeding relationship.

I think a big part of my pain is from people trying hard to comfort me with comments like fed is best. That didn't help and it made me feel like my feelings were invalid. All I wanted was for people to listen and acknowledge my struggle without outside opinions or advice – unless explicitly asked.

Funnily enough, what women felt was really important was when people actually stopped and asked how they were and really listened. A lot of mothers felt a great degree of comfort if they were given the chance to talk about their experiences and how they felt at having to stop. They felt acknowledged. Seen. Validated. And like they mattered – as more than a carrier of and carer for their baby. As the saying goes, when a baby is born, so is a mother. And her emotions and wellbeing matter.

6. Consider how those who need to formula feed are practically supported

More kindness. More compassion. Less damnation for bottles. Fewer breast is best posters. Just be accepting.

This is really important, and came out clearly in women's stories. Somehow, many women seemed to fall through the gaps of infant feeding care and support when they started using formula. So many women repeated the tale that once they stopped breastfeeding, any support they were getting seemed to fall away. They weren't told how to make up a bottle of formula correctly (which is an important part of ensuring formula is prepared safely), how to pace feed or how much milk to give their baby. It was somehow assumed that because there were instructions on the side of the tin, that was all that was needed.

> *More support for non-breastfeeding mums. I feel like it's only the breastfeeding mums who get support and the bottle/ formula-feeding mums are forgotten/ignored and made to feel like they are doing something wrong. There are lactation consultants for breastfeeding mums, but who do formula feeding mums go to for support and help?*

Something is going wrong here. Years ago, the message about not promoting formula to pregnant women got a bit confused. Some midwives were saying that they weren't allowed to mention it at all, and to always assume women were breastfeeding, and if they were asked how to make up formula they had to refuse. Somehow the Baby Friendly Initiative got mixed up with this and some health professionals were saying that if their area was Baby Friendly accredited they couldn't give any information or support for formula-feeding at all.

This is just not true. The Baby Friendly Initiative[5] and other government-linked campaign/information sources[6] such as Start for Life publish information online and in print on how to make up formula for your baby. Women should have been directed towards it.

There is a major difference between promoting formula and supporting women with formula-feeding if that's what they decide to do. Proper support provides a standard of care to all women, and helps women feel less like they are being ignored because they are not breastfeeding. And besides all of that, accurate information on how to feed responsively, make up a bottle and not overfeed plays an important role in reducing the risks associated with formula, such as incorrect bottle preparation or overfeeding.

Women also wanted to see far more information on mixed feeding. Combining breast and formula-feeding seems to be a bit of a mystery, doesn't it? It comes up time and time again when I talk to mothers about their experiences of stopping breastfeeding – the fact that no one spoke to them about mixed feeding. Somehow, when they were struggling and wanting to use formula, everyone assumed that it was all over and they might as well just exclusively formula feed.

> *The complete lack of support and information around mixed feeding alienates a lot of women. If mixed feeding was more supported as an option I'm sure women would carry on.*

Lots of mothers talked about the fact that breastfeeding seemed to be presented as an either/or decision, and this has cropped up in other research.[7] They felt that information and support messages were based around a gold standard of breastfeeding exclusively, and that mothers who could not meet that standard were not supported. If they asked about giving a bottle of formula while struggling, they were told that this would damage their supply. When they wanted to stop breastfeeding, no one talked them through whether they wanted to stop breastfeeding or whether they wanted to use formula – and there is a big difference there. When women did 'crack', as they described it, and gave formula, they felt guilty, as if they had 'ruined things' and it was all over.

We know from research that the greatest protection of babies' health comes from exclusive breastfeeding, and that supplementing can be a gamble when it comes to milk supply.

But there is also plenty of research that shows it's a continuum, with partial breastfeeding (mixed feeding) showing benefits as well. Saying that if you can't exclusively breastfeed you might as well stop is similar to saying that if you can't eat five fruit and veg a day you might as well not eat any. Or if you can't run 10k, there's no point even going for a walk. Most things in life aren't so black and white, but for many women their experience was that breastfeeding was presented that way.

Supplementing doesn't necessarily have to be the end of breastfeeding. If mums need to supplement, let them know they can continue breastfeeding and support them to keep their supply up.

Another idea highlighted was that greater recognition was needed for women who met or exceeded their own goals, particularly in challenging situations, even though this might not be as long as health guidelines would promote. Recognising the achievement of those who fell outside this would help women to feel that they had achieved something or overcome barriers, and send a wider message that breastfeeding wasn't just for women who could do so exclusively for a long time. Women felt that they were made to feel like failures for not meeting these set goals, when initially they were happy with what they achieved.

I didn't feel that bad when I first stopped breastfeeding because I was quite unsure of it in the first place and promised myself I would give it a go and do it for a couple of weeks or so to let her get that first goodness. But then I managed to keep going for a bit longer and did six weeks for her in the end. I was pretty chuffed as that was longer than most people I know managed. But then everyone I met kept trying to console me or tell me it didn't matter or asking what went wrong. But nothing went wrong, I breastfed for longer than I ever thought I could? But them going on and on at me gradually made me feel worried and guilty over time. Could I have tried harder? Was it really not that good after all? I do worry.

Another idea was to make sure that there were more options for mothers who were formula-feeding to attend feeding support groups. Many felt that there were only groups for breastfeeding mothers, particularly those who exclusively breastfed, and they were unsure where to turn for guidance. Others simply wanted the social support, but all their friends went along to feeding groups and they couldn't go.

Offer more support networks for bottle-feeding mums too. In my area there's breastfeeding groups and I used to enjoy going but once I started bottle-feeding I felt isolated and there's no other free groups to attend.

Some suggested that having at least a few mixed feeding group options might help others change their mind about breastfeeding future babies, especially if they hadn't really been exposed to breastfeeding before – which may be an unintended consequence of breastfeeding-only groups. Those who rarely see it, are even less likely to do it.

Support mums both ways. A baby group where women breast and bottle-feed can lead to women who bottle-feed their first considering breast on second when they talk about experience.

Another interesting idea was whether there could be some system in place, perhaps a sticker on notes, in the red book, or on the computer system, to stop every health professional asking about feeding. This makes sense. We know that trauma is more likely if you keep being reminded of the event over and over, and at each health appointment women were being asked again how they were feeding and having to recall the experience.

Every time I went for an appointment I got asked how I was feeding him and then invariably why. I did not want to keep repeating my story, or how I felt – justifying it. It hurt and brought everything back up as I wondered whether they were judging me or making decisions based on the type of mum I thought they thought I was.

7. Value mothers more

One of the core ideas women raised was that if we just focused away from feeding for a moment, and looked instead at how we could support mothers more broadly, perhaps we wouldn't have such issues with breastfeeding grief in the first place. If mothers (and women) were better valued and supported they would be less likely to have breastfeeding difficulties, and if they did they would be supported and nurtured through any feelings if they needed to stop.

Mothering, infant feeding and mental health are closely intertwined, as we have seen throughout this book. If a woman is struggling in one area, it is likely the others will be affected. For some women, mental health challenges will be more complex and present before she has had her baby. For others they are a consequence of mothering in a society that doesn't really support them.[8]

We know that when mothers are listened to and cared for, their mental health is better. But our society continues to let new mothers down by not seeing their challenges and not valuing the physical and emotional work that they do every day. We must increase our investment in supporting new families, raising their value, and ensuring that they have a network of support around them.

Breastfeeding in the early weeks is a full-time job in itself. We should recognise this and help new mothers like they do in other countries so that they can get on with feeding and taking care of themselves and not have to do everything else. Women end up bottle-feeding as they think at least the baby can be fed by someone else and that's one less thing to do.

How many times do you hear or see this story? Where is the valuing and recognition of what new mothers do? How many people really know how to help a new mother and come and do so – and how many just excitedly ask to come round and visit and then sit there and hog the baby? How do we get society to understand that when a baby is born, so is a mother, and she needs just as much gentle care and attention as the baby?

How many times is a woman's ability to breastfeed damaged by needing to return to work? Increasing maternity leave and pay not only supports women by giving them the option of spending more time at home with their baby, but also sends a clear message that motherhood is valued.

In the UK we have maternity leave and pay protection, but unless your employer offers enhanced support, the level of pay drops significantly after six weeks to a level many cannot survive on for long. In the USA there is still no statutory leave at all. Yet in Scandinavia, where breastfeeding rates are high, maternity leave policies allow for far longer at home. In Sweden, mothers are entitled to 15 months leave at 90% pay (and are then supported through a whole range of family-friendly working policies and subsidised childcare).[9]

8. Create a society that values human milk

The final idea raised by women in the research was to ensure that women's breastfeeding experiences and wellbeing were not being affected by an industry designed to make profit from every woman who stops breastfeeding. Some women reported that they could see the formula industry deliberately targeting mothers and health professionals in all these different ways, which they felt made breastfeeding much more difficult for women.

The formula industry deliberately stirs up how I and many other women feel just to cause tension and sell more products. They have to be stopped.

It is against UK law to promote products aimed at replacing breastmilk for babies under six months old for a reason. Families do not need the interference of industry in their decisions on infant feeding. This is not an anti-formula statement: formula is needed for babies who cannot be breastfed as they cannot thrive on cows' milk alone. However, the formula industry in the UK spends over US$9 billion a year deliberately marketing their products at parents.[10]

How babies are fed is too important a decision to be influenced by marketing. If a mother is breastfeeding she does not need to have formula promoted to her. If a mother needs or chooses to use formula, then it is vital that her baby gets the best possible product – as it is not just food, but a specialist product that her baby would suffer without.

Mothers also raised the idea that we should expand access to donor human milk for more babies.

We must start talking more about the possibility of opening up breast milk banks to all.

Although the idea that every woman who does not breastfeed could simply access donor human milk (DHM) instead of infant formula is probably far-fetched, I would certainly like to see greater access for women in specific situations.

DHM is currently typically available for only the most premature and sickest babies, usually born before 32 weeks, if their mother cannot produce sufficient milk herself. DHM can be lifesaving for these babies, reducing their risk of developing complications of prematurity such as necrotising enterocolitis; reducing their stay in hospital; and acting as a 'bridge' to help their mothers establish their own milk supply.[8]

Although we couldn't open up access to all, increasing DHM in specific situations would help offer women more choices. What if we could offer it to women who cannot breastfeed because of having had a mastectomy, or who are undergoing chemotherapy? What if older babies who are seriously unwell and struggle to tolerate other foods could be given it?

And what if those babies whose mothers are struggling to make enough milk of their own in the early days, but who really want to avoid formula, could have the option of human milk instead? Research has suggested that very small amounts of formula milk, given via a syringe, do not have an impact on breastfeeding continuation (although more research is needed), which is great.[11] But what if DHM was available instead, in very small amounts, for women who needed to do this and did not want to use formula? In the study above that used very small amounts of formula, just 10ml was used a few times a day for around two days. Around 100ml of DHM only costs about £15.[10]

These things are a very real possibility and the Human Milk Foundation is a charity dedicated to raising money to enable more babies in these situations to have access to DHM. You can read more about their work and some of the stories of families who have benefited, here: www.humanmilkfoundation.org.

For example, Shurron Rosales's son Koan received donor human milk when he was born with a genetic neurological condition and spent most of his first two months in intensive care. Koan needed to be fed through a tube in his early days meaning Shurron needed to express milk regularly for him. Exhausted from birth and traumatised by everything Koan was going through meant that Shurron didn't have enough milk in those early days, but she really wanted Koan to have an exclusive breastmilk diet.

The family were lucky enough to be able to receive a five-week supply of donor milk from the Hearts Milk Bank, meaning that while Shurron could continue to encourage her breastmilk supply, the pressure was reduced and Koan could have an exclusive breastmilk diet. With the support of the milk bank and time Koan was soon exclusively breastfed and was breastfed for over two years.

Shurron explained what donor milk meant to her:

I knew breastmilk would give my newborn son, who had so much going against him health-wise, a fighting chance at getting stronger and create the building blocks to a healthier tomorrow. It also meant I could feel like I was fulfilling my role as a mother. So much was out of my control when he was in hospital in his first few months and more than ever when he was given a life-changing diagnosis. This finally felt like something I could do for him. I fought for him to have donor milk, and it gave me a sense of achievement and purpose as a mother I thought I'd lost when we couldn't establish breastfeeding at first.

Going on to re-establish breastfeeding meant we could bond, and start to stitch back together the wounds that I felt tore me apart in those early days. It meant I could give him the perfect tailor-made food and antibodies that he needed on demand. It meant he could use his mouth to feed (rather than being fed through a tube) and learn skills that I believe set him up for success with feeding and will help him with his speech. Breastmilk – and those early days of donor milk supplementation – meant the world to my son, to me and to my family.

Finally, central to all of this must be helping women through their grief and supporting them in realising that it is not their fault. If they wanted to breastfeed and it was important to them and they couldn't, then it is highly likely that they have stopped feeding either because of a physiological issue outside of their control, or because of trying to breastfeed in a society and network that just did not support them to do so. In the words of Baby Friendly UK:

We need to change the conversation around breastfeeding by stopping laying the responsibility for this major public health issue in the laps of individual women and acknowledging the role that politics and society has to play at every level.

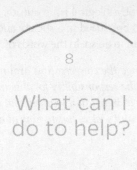

8

What can I do to help?

If you are feeling inspired to help us change the world, there are a number of things you can do:

- Sign our Better breastfeeding campaign to end cuts to breastfeeding support bit.ly/2TazA3d.
- Sign the Baby Friendly UK Call to Action, calling on governments to take steps to enable women to breastfeed for longer www.unicef.org.uk/babyfriendly/about/call-to-action.
- Write to your local MP and ask them to attend meetings of the All Party Parliamentary Group (APPG) on Infant Feeding and Inequalities chaired by Alison Thewliss MP
- Check out the work of 'Human milk' – an organisation dedicated to spreading awareness of how human milk protects mothers and babies. They have resources that can be used to support students and in education www.human-milk.com.
- Support the work of the charity Baby Milk Action, which fights tirelessly to stop industry from breaking

the International Code of Marketing of Breastmilk
Substitutes www.babymilkaction.org.

- If you or someone you support is interested in
donating their milk, details of local milk banks are at
www.ukamb.org/milk-banks. At present, the Hearts
Milk Bank (www.heartsmilkbank.org), just north
of London, is the only milk bank that will recruit
mothers with babies older than six months, but this
may change in the near future.

- For more information on breastfeeding and mental
health, look up the work of the Maternal Mental
Health Alliance. In collaboration with a wide range
of infant feeding and maternal mental health experts,
they have recently produced a perinatal mental
health competency framework for professionals and
volunteers who support infant feeding bit.ly/2Vy8eAM.
The Royal College of General Practitioners also has
a useful protocol called *Infant feeding: Wellbeing and
maternal mental health* bit.ly/2TujoJh.

- For more inspiration for change in the world of birth
and babies look to the Positive Birth Movement,
Association for Improvement in Maternity Services
(AIMS), the Association for Radical Midwives (ARM)
and *The Roar Behind the Silence* book. For more
information check out the All4Maternity page www.
all4birth.com.

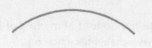

Acknowledgements

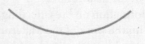

There are three groups of people I must thank for making this book happen.

First – my family, who have come to not even bat an eyelid when I casually mention 'So… thing is… *I've had another book idea*'. This includes my Pinter & Martin family, who equally have simply come to say '*Lovely… when can you do it by?*'

Second – the mothers who helped by telling me their stories. Either directly in my research, in passing conversations, or in the countless stories we see every day that say the same thing: women are still being failed. I know it is not easy to share your grief. Often therapeutic and cathartic, yes. But not easy. Never easy. We are all so grateful.

Third – anyone who has ever written a media story writing off women's emotions as simply a consequence of 'pressure to breastfeed', or bullied or mocked them without considering the real story behind women's grief. Your countless attempts to pretend that breastfeeding isn't important to many women have had an impact. I thank you too.

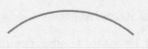

References

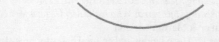

Chapter 1: Why does breastfeeding matter so much to women?

1. Brown A, Lee M 'An exploration of the attitudes and experiences of mothers in the United Kingdom who chose to breastfeed exclusively for 6 months postpartum'. *Breastfeeding Medicine*. 2011 Aug 1;6(4):197-204.

2. Kent JC, et al. 'Principles for maintaining or increasing breast milk production'. *JOGNN*. 2012 Jan 1;41(1):114-21.

3. Chowdhury R et al. 'Breastfeeding and maternal health outcomes: a systematic review and meta-analysis'. *Acta Paediatrica*. 2015 Dec;104:96-113.

4. www.independent.co.uk/life-style/health-and-families/health-news/viagra-number-of-prescriptions-for-erectile-dysfunction-drugs-rises-by-more-than-a-quarter-10372318.html

5. www.independent.co.uk/news/science/pms-erectile-dysfunction-studies-penis-problems-period-pre-menstrual-pains-science-disparity-a7198681.html

6. Latini, D et al. 'Psychological impact of erectile dysfunction: validation of a new health related quality of life measure for patients with erectile dysfunction'. *The Journal of Urology* 2002: 168(5), pp.2086-2091.

7. Jung C *Lactivism: How feminists and fundamentalists, hippies and yuppies, and physicians and politicians made breastfeeding big business and bad policy*. Basic Books; 2015 Nov 24.

8. Schmied, V and Lupton, D, 2001. 'Blurring the boundaries:

breastfeeding and maternal subjectivity'. *Sociology of Health & Illness*, 23(2), pp.234-250.

9. Marshall JL et al. 'Being a 'good mother': managing breastfeeding and merging identities'. *Social Science & Medicine*. 2007 Nov 1;65(10):2147-59.

10. Flacking R et al. 'Trustful bonds: a key to "becoming a mother" and to reciprocal breastfeeding. Stories of mothers of very preterm infants at a neonatal unit'. *Social Science & Medicine*. 2006 Jan 1;62(1):70-80.

11. Kendall-Tackett K et al. 'Depression, sleep quality, and maternal well-being in postpartum women with a history of sexual assault: A comparison of breastfeeding, mixed-feeding, and formula-feeding mothers'. *Breastfeeding Medicine*. 2013 Feb 1;8(1):16-22.

12. Brown A *Breastfeeding Uncovered: Who really decides how we feed our babies?* 2016. Pinter & Martin: London

13. Laroia N, Sharma D 'The religious and cultural bases for breastfeeding practices among the Hindus'. *Breastfeeding Medicine*. 2006 Jun 1;1(2):94-8.

14. Shaikh, U and Ahmed, O, 2006. 'Islam and infant feeding'. *Breastfeeding Medicine*, 1(3), pp.164-167.

15. Salmon, M, 1994. 'The cultural significance of breastfeeding and infant care in early modern England and America'. *Journal of Social History*, pp.247-269.

16. Shaw R. 'Performing breastfeeding: embodiment, ethics and the maternal subject'. *Feminist Review*. 2004 Nov 1;78(1):99-116.

Chapter 2: How do women feel when they are unable to meet their breastfeeding goals?

1. Labbok, M, 2008 'Exploration of guilt among mothers who do not breastfeed: the physician's role'. *Journal of Human Lactation*, 24(1), 80-84.

2. Thomson, G, Ebisch-Burton, K, and Flacking, R, 2015. 'Shame if you do–shame if you don't: women's experiences of infant feeding'. *Maternal & Child Nutrition*, 11(1), 33-46.

3. Brown A. 'What Do Women Lose if They Are Prevented From Meeting Their Breastfeeding Goals?'. *Clinical Lactation*. 2018 Nov 1;9(4):200-7.

4. Lee EJ 'Living with risk in the age of 'intensive motherhood': Maternal identity and infant feeding'. *Health, Risk & Society*. 2008 Oct 1;10(5):467-77.

5. Blaine B, Crocker J 'Self-esteem and self-serving biases in reactions to positive and negative events: An integrative review'. In *Self-esteem*

1993 (pp. 55-85). Springer, Boston, MA.
6. Victora CG et al 'Breastfeeding in the 21st century: epidemiology, mechanisms, and lifelong effect'. *The Lancet*. 2016 Jan 30;387(10017):475-90.

Chapter 3: Breastfeeding, stopping breastfeeding and the risk of postnatal depression

1. Shields SA 'The politics of emotion in everyday life: "Appropriate" emotion and claims on identity'. *Review of General Psychology*. 2005 Mar;9(1):3-15.
2. Holland JM et al. 'The underlying structure of grief: A taxometric investigation of prolonged and normal reactions to loss'. *Journal of Psychopathology and Behavioral Assessment*. 2009 Sep 1;31(3):190-201.
3. Dennis CL, McQueen K 'The relationship between infant-feeding outcomes and postpartum depression: a qualitative systematic review'. *Pediatrics*. 2009 Apr 1;123(4):e736-51.
4. Borra C et al. 2015. 'New evidence on breastfeeding and postpartum depression: the importance of understanding women's intentions'. *Maternal and Child Health Journal*, 19(4), 897-907.
5. Brown, A et al. 2016. 'Understanding the relationship between breastfeeding and postnatal depression: the role of pain and physical difficulties'. *Journal of Advanced Nursing*, 72(2), 273-282.
6. Rudzik AE et al. 'Discrepancies in maternal reports of infant sleep vs. actigraphy by mode of feeding'. *Sleep Medicine*. 2018 Sep 1;49:90-8.
7. Engler A et al. 2012. 'Breastfeeding may improve nocturnal sleep and reduce infantile colic: potential role of breast milk melatonin'. *European Journal of Pediatrics*, 171(4), 729-732.
8. Blyton, D et al. 2002. 'Lactation is associated with an increase in slow-wave sleep in women'. *Journal of Sleep Research*, 11(4), 297-303.
9. Cong Z et al. 'The Effect of Feeding Method on Sleep Duration, Maternal Wellbeing, and Pospartum Depression'. *Clinical Lactation*. 2011;2(2):22-6.
10. Kendall-Tackett K 'A new paradigm for depression in new mothers: the central role of inflammation and how breastfeeding and anti-inflammatory treatments protect maternal mental health'. *International Breastfeeding Journal*. 2007 Mar;2(1):6.
11. Groër MW et al. 'Immunity, inflammation and infection in post-partum breast and formula feeders'. *American Journal of Reproductive Immunology*. 2005, 54: 222-231
12. Brown A. 'What Do Women Lose if They Are Prevented From Meeting Their Breastfeeding Goals?'. *Clinical Lactation*. 2018 Nov

1;9(4):200-7.

13. IsHak WW et al. 'Pain and depression: A systematic review'. *Harvard Review of Psychiatry*. 2018 Nov 1;26(6):352-63.

14. Ahmed AH et al. 'Relationship between sleep quality, depression symptoms, and blood glucose in pregnant women'. *Western Journal of Nursing Research*. 2018 Nov 8:0193945918809714.

15. Scotland M *Why Postnatal Depression Matters*. 2015 Pinter & Martin Ltd.

16. Laroia N, Sharma D 'The religious and cultural bases for breastfeeding practices among the Hindus'. *Breastfeeding Medicine*. 2006 Jun 1;1(2):94-8.

Chapter 4: Can not being able to breastfeed cause psychological trauma?

1. American Psychiatric Association. (2013) Diagnostic and statistical manual of mental disorders, (5th ed.). Washington, DC: Author.

2. icd.who.int/browse10/2016/en#/F43.1

3. Beck, CT 2009. 'Birth trauma and its sequelae'. *Journal of Trauma & Dissociation*, 10(2), 189-203.

4. Brown A, Jordan S 'Impact of birth complications on breastfeeding duration: an internet survey'. *Journal of Advanced Nursing*. 2013 Apr;69(4):828-39.

5. Beck CT, Watson S 'Subsequent childbirth after a previous traumatic birth'. *Nursing Research*. 2010 Jul 1;59(4):241-9.

6. Harris R, Ayers S 'What makes labour and birth traumatic? A survey of intrapartum 'hotspots''. *Psychology & Health*. 2012 Oct 1;27(10):1166-77.

7. Beck CT, Watson S 'Subsequent childbirth after a previous traumatic birth'. *Nursing Research*. 2010 Jul 1;59(4):241-9.

8. McClellan HL et al. 'Nipple pain during breastfeeding with or without visible trauma'. *Journal of Human Lactation*. 2012 Nov;28(4):511-21.

9. Andersen LB et al. 'Risk factors for developing post-traumatic stress disorder following childbirth: a systematic review'. *Acta Obstetricia et Gynecologica Scandinavica*. 2012 Nov;91(11):1261-72.

10. www.centreformentalhealth.org.uk/blog/centre-mental-health-blog/what-happened-you-how-health-care-can-become-trauma-informed

11. www.nhs.uk/oneyou/for-your-mind/possible-causes#possible-causes-what-affects-mental-health

12. www.integration.samhsa.gov/clinical-practice/trauma

13. Pearlman LA, Saakvitne KW *Trauma and the therapist: Countertransference and vicarious traumatization in psychotherapy*

with incest survivors. WW Norton & Co; 1995.

14. Allen JG *Coping with trauma: A guide to self-understanding.* American Psychiatric Association; 1995.

15. Ehlers A, Clark DM 'A cognitive model of posttraumatic stress disorder'. *Behaviour Research And Therapy.* 2000 Apr 1;38(4):319-45.

16. Svanberg E *Why Birth Trauma Matters.* 2019, Pinter and Martin Ltd.

Chapter 5: Why do so many women struggle to breastfeed?

1. McAndrew F et al. 2012. 'Infant feeding survey 2010'. *Leeds: Health and Social Care Information Centre.*

2. Victora CG et al. 2016. 'Breastfeeding in the 21st century: epidemiology, mechanisms, and lifelong effect'. *The Lancet,* 387(10017):475-490.

3. Huggins K et al. 'Markers of lactation insufficiency: a study of 34 mothers'. *Current Issues in Clinical Lactation.* 2000;1:25-35.

4. Souto GC et al. 'The impact of breast reduction surgery on breastfeeding performance'. *Journal of Human Lactation.* 2003 Feb;19(1):43-9.

5. Amir LH 'Breastfeeding: managing 'supply' difficulties'. *Australian Family Physician.* 2006 Sep;35(9):686.

6. Lawrence RM and Lawrence RA 2001. 'Given the benefits of breastfeeding, what contraindications exist?' *Pediatric Clinics,* 48(1):235-251.

7. Bosire R et al. 'High rates of exclusive breastfeeding in both arms of a peer counseling study promoting EBF among HIV-infected Kenyan women'. *Breastfeeding Medicine.* 2016 Mar 1;11(2):56-63.

8. Jones W *Breastfeeding and Medication.* Routledge; 2018 May 11.

9. Brown A et al. 'A lifeline when no one else wants to give you an answer. An evaluation of the Drugs in Breastmilk service. *Breastfeeding Network.*

10. www.theguardian.com/lifeandstyle/2018/jul/27/breastfeeding-support-services-failing-mothers-due-to-cuts

11. McClellan et al. 'Nipple pain during breastfeeding with or without visible trauma'. *Journal of Human Lactation.* 2012 Nov;28(4):511-21.

12. Brown, A et al. 2016. 'Understanding the relationship between breastfeeding and postnatal depression: the role of pain and physical difficulties'. *Journal of Advanced Nursing,* 72(2), 273-282.

13. Brown A *Breastfeeding Uncovered: Who really decides how we feed our babies?* 2016. Pinter & Martin Ltd.

14. Daly SE, Hartmann PE 'Infant demand and milk supply. Part 1: Infant demand and milk production in lactating women'. *Journal of Human*

Lactation. 1995 Mar;11(1):21-6.

15. Brown A, Arnott B 'Breastfeeding duration and early parenting behaviour: the importance of an infant-led, responsive style'. *PloS One*. 2014 Feb 12;9(2):e83893.

16. Cusk, R. (2014). *A Life's Work*. Faber & Faber.

17. Darwent, K et al. 2016. 'The Infant Feeding Genogram: a tool for exploring family infant feeding history and identifying support needs'. *BMC Pregnancy and Childbirth*, 16(1): 315.

18. Bäckström CA et al. 'Two sides of breastfeeding support: experiences of women and midwives'. *International Breastfeeding Journal*. 2010 Dec;5(1):20.

19. Trickey H et al. 2017. 'Nain, Mam and Me: Historical artefacts as prompts for reminiscence, reflection and conversation about feeding babies. A qualitative development study'. *Research for All*, 1(1):64-83.

20. Walker K 2017. 'What issues do lesbian co-mothers face in their transition to parenthood?' *NCT Perspectives*, 34

21. Brown A & Davies R 2014. 'Fathers' experiences of supporting breastfeeding: challenges for breastfeeding promotion and education'. *Maternal & Child Nutrition*, 10(4):510-526.

22. Maternity Action UK 2018 maternityaction.org.uk

23. Gatrell CJ 2007. 'Secrets and lies breastfeeding and professional paid work'. *Social Science and Medicine*, 65(2): 393-404.

24. Donnelly A, Snowden HH, Renfrew MJ 2000. 'Commercial hospital discharge packs for breastfeeding women'. *Cochrane Database of Systematic Reviews*, (2).

25. Berry NJ, Jones SC and Iverson D 2012. 'Toddler milk advertising in Australia: Infant formula advertising in disguise?' *Australasian Marketing Journal*, 20(1): 24-27.

26. Allers KS. *The big letdown: How medicine, big business, and feminism undermine breastfeeding*. St. Martin's Press; 2017 Jan 24.

Chapter 6: Healing from your own breastfeeding experience

1. Labbok M 2008. 'Exploration of guilt among mothers who do not breastfeed: the physician's role'. *Journal of Human Lactation*, 24(1), 80-84.

2. Kübler-Ross E, Kessler D *On grief and grieving: Finding the meaning of grief through the five stages of loss*. Simon and Schuster; 2005.

3. Svanberg E *Why Birth Trauma Matters*. 2019. Pinter and Martin Ltd.

4. www.helpguide.org/articles/ptsd-trauma/coping-with-emotional-and-psychological-trauma.htm

5. www.rcpsych.ac.uk/mental-health/problems-disorders/coping-after-a-traumatic-event

6. www.svri.org/sites/default/files/attachments/2016-01-13/HADS.pdf

7. Bastos MH et al. 'Debriefing interventions for the prevention of psychological trauma in women following childbirth'. *Cochrane Database of Systematic Reviews*. 2015(4).

8. Seidler GH, Wagner FE 'Comparing the efficacy of EMDR and trauma-focused cognitive-behavioral therapy in the treatment of PTSD: a meta-analytic study'. *Psychological Medicine*. 2006 Nov;36(11):1515-22.

Chapter 7: What can we do to make things better?

1. Brown A et al. 'A lifeline when no one else wants to give you an answer. An evaluation of the Drugs in Breastmilk service'. *Breastfeeding Network*.

2. Grayson L *Unlatched: the evolution of breastfeeding and the marketing of a controversy*. Harper Collins.

3. WBTI (2016). *World Breastfeeding Trends Initiative UK Report*. ukbreastfeedingtrends.files.wordpress.com/2017/03/wbti-uk-report-2016-part-1-14-2-17.pdf

4. Greene J et al. 'Feeding preferences and attitudes to breastfeeding and its promotion among teenagers in Northern Ireland'. *Journal of Human Lactation*. 2003 Feb;19(1):57-65.

5. www.unicef.org.uk/babyfriendly/baby-friendly-resources/bottle-feeding-resources/guide-to-bottle-feeding/

6. campaignresources.phe.gov.uk/resources/campaigns/2/resources/232

7. Brown A 2016. 'What do women really want? Lessons for breastfeeding promotion and education'. *Breastfeeding Medicine*, 11(3): 102-110.

8. McMahon M *Why Mothering Matters*. 2019. Pinter & Martin Ltd.

9. www.oecd.org/els/soc/PF2_1_Parental_leave_systems.pdf; www.savethechildren.org.uk/content/dam/gb/reports/health/dont-push-it.pdf

10. www.huffingtonpost.co.uk/entry/donor-human-milk_uk_5c0422d8e4b024223b60af12

11. Flaherman VJ, Aby J, Burgos AE, Lee KA, Cabana MD, Newman TB. Effect of early limited formula on duration and exclusivity of breastfeeding in at-risk infants: an RCT. Pediatrics. 2013 Jun 1;131(6):1059-65.

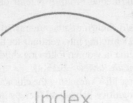

Index

Series editor: Susan Last

pinterandmartin.com